Wonderful Pregnancy

Pregnancy Questions and Answers from Experts

Wonderful Pregnancy

Pregnancy Questions and Answers from Experts

Howard E. Herrell, MD, FACOG
Antonia K. Roberts, MD, FACOG
Hosts of *Thinking About OB/GYN* Podcast

www.wonderfulpregnancy.com

With contributions from Bonnie Buckles, MD, and Madeline White, DO.

Sonic Elephant

First Edition.

Medicine is a vibrant and ever-changing discipline. The information provided within this book is for general educational purposes only. While we try to keep the information up-to-date and correct, there are no representations or warranties, express or implied, about the completeness, accuracy, reliability, suitability, or availability with respect to the information, products, techniques, or related graphics contained in this book for any purpose. Any use of this information is at your own risk.

The indications and dosages of all drugs in the book have been recommended in the medical literature and conform to the practices of the general medical community. The medications described do not necessarily have specific approval by the Food and Drug Administration for use in the diseases and dosages for which they are recommended. The package insert for each drug should be consulted for use and dosage as approved by the FDA. Because standards of usage change, it is advisable to keep abreast of revised recommendations, particularly those concerning new drugs.

Published by Sonic Elephant
www.sonicelephant.com

ISBN: 978-0-9993696-2-3

10 9 8 7 6 5 4 3 2 1

Contents

Getting Started

How do we get this thing started?

If you're not pregnant already, you may have a few questions about getting the show on the road. If you are pregnant already, congratulations and skip this chapter!

How long does it take after stopping birth control to get pregnant?

This depends on the birth control method you use and how your body responds. If you have an IUD removed, it is possible for you to become pregnant the first cycle after its removal. Since IUDs don't normally affect ovulation, it is possible to become pregnant just a few days after removal. The same goes for NEXPLANON, the arm rod contraceptive. Once the rod is removed, you can become pregnant within the first cycle.

If you take the combination birth control pill, which contains both estrogen and progesterone, or a progesterone-only pill, you can become pregnant also within the first cycle, as ovulation will resume within the month after you stop the pill, and your cervical mucus will return to normal rapidly. About 40% of progesterone-only pill users still regularly ovulate, which is why it is important not to miss doses while trying to prevent pregnancy with that method. Remember, the primary pregnancy prevention mechanism of the progesterone-only pill is like that of the progestin IUDs or implants - they thicken the cervical mucus.

Your chance of becoming pregnant in any given month of trying is around 20% or less, even if everything is normal. So, it's not likely that you'll become pregnant right after stopping birth control, but it is possible, and you don't need to stop birth control until right before you would like to become pregnant. In some cases, your menses might not resume after stopping these forms of birth control and that's not likely due to the birth control, but to an underlying ovulation or fertility problem. If your periods don't become normal after stopping any of these methods of birth control within two or three months, you should see your doctor. Even if everything is working well, it still can take several months for the average couple to get pregnant. If you've tried for a year without success (or six months, if you're over the age of 35), you should see your doctor for a fertility evaluation.

When you stop the Depo-Provera shot, however, you may not have an immediate return to fertility. This is one of the down sides of the shot. It can take some women several months or even well over a year for ovulation to return. The contraceptive effect of each shot lasts reliably for 12-15 weeks, which is why we recommend that patients get the shot every three months. Some patients choose to stop the Depo-Provera shot six months or more in advance of a planned pregnancy to avoid an unnecessary delay in conception.

Barrier methods such as condoms or the diaphragm, when they are not used, allow for the possibility of immediate conception if you ovulate regularly. Remember, becoming pregnant may take up to a year even if there are no issues. Don't get discouraged if it takes a while and make sure you are talking with your doctor throughout the process if you are worried about anything or suspect something is wrong, especially if your menses aren't regular.

When is the best time to have sex to get pregnant?

Sex just before the time of ovulation is the best way to achieve pregnancy. The optimal time to have sex is during the five days leading up to the day of ovulation. Daily sex is fine but having sex at least every other day in your "fertile window" is ideal. The absolute best day is the day right before ovulation, so if you are tracking your ovulation timing, make sure you include that day for intercourse.

How can I determine when I'm ovulating?

Ovulation occurs 14 days before the first day of your next period. For women with a "typical" 28-day menstrual cycle, this means ovulation occurs on cycle day 14, where the first day of bleeding is day 1. However, not all women have a 28-day cycle. If you have a 30-day cycle, ovulation will occur on day 16 (30 minus 14) or if you have a 26-day cycle, it will occur on day 12 (26 minus 14).

Some clues that you may be ovulating include a thicker, sticky cervical mucus (resembling egg whites) or a change in basal body temperature (prior to ovulation, basal body temperature measured first thing in the morning declines slightly and immediately after ovulation it rises again). These signs are not always accurate and can be difficult to assess. Cervical mucus and body temperature are subject to wide variation from person to person.

Over-the-counter ovulation detection kits can be purchased that are much better at determining ovulation. These urine tests are used with the first urination of the day, and they detect the surge in luteinizing hormone (LH) that occurs the day before ovulation. These are not always accurate but are much better than basal body temperature or cervical mucus monitoring and they have the benefit of determining ovulation the day before, which is an ideal day to have sex when trying to become pregnant.

If your cycle is irregular, if it is longer than 35 days, or if it is shorter than 21 days, talk to your doctor about how you can determine when you are ovulating, or if you need an evaluation to make sure you are ovulating. We can test your blood for a surge of progesterone about 8 days after the suspected day of ovulation to confirm that you ovulated. If you did not, there are medical treatments to help you ovulate.

Should I have a preconception visit?

These are not always necessary, but they can certainly be helpful! If there are factors in your medical or family history that you think might make getting pregnant more difficult or complicate a pregnancy, then your doctor can discuss these with you and give you advice and help optimize your health before becoming pregnant.

If you have chronic medical problems like diabetes, hypertension, or other conditions that require you to take medication, a preconception visit is a great idea. Getting medical conditions optimally managed with safe medications is the goal.

Should I stop any of my medications?

Don't stop your medications until you discuss them with your doctor! Most medications are perfectly safe to take throughout pregnancy. Others may be stopped, but we often have alternative treatments that can be used to manage your medical conditions.

Do I need to take a prenatal vitamin before becoming pregnant?

Yes! In fact, taking the prenatal vitamin before becoming pregnant is ideal. Building levels of folic acid in your body helps to reduce the risk of neural tube defects and some studies show that women who take a prenatal vitamin in the months leading up to conception have less nausea and vomiting in the first trimester of pregnancy.

You don't need anything fancy. A basic prenatal vitamin is more than enough; try to take this for at least three months before conceiving. In 2023, the U.S. Government Accountability Office tested twelve different undisclosed prenatal vitamin brands and found that eleven of them did not contain nutrients in the amounts claimed on their labels. This included brands boasting "third-party testing." They have recommended more FDA oversight into nutritional supplements such as prenatal vitamins, which are currently considered a "food" instead of medication and are not regulated in the same way as medications.

Do I need any vaccinations before pregnancy?

The most important vaccine that you should get prior to pregnancy is the MMR (measles, mumps, rubella) vaccine. Many people received this vaccine during their childhood; however, immunity can wane over time. Your doctor can order a blood test called a titer that looks at your immunity to those diseases and will decide based on your antibody levels whether you should get the vaccine series again (usually two doses 28 days apart). Historically, congenital rubella syndrome was a devastating disease that affected newborns whose mothers developed rubella in the first trimester. Thankfully, because of the vaccine, this condition is now rare with fewer than 1,000 cases a year but even those are preventable.

I'm Pregnant!?!

Yay! You're pregnant! So, what's next?

Planned or unplanned, whether it's your first or your fifth, pregnancy is exciting and nerve-wracking at the same time. When you're pregnant, everyone has an opinion about what you should and shouldn't do. The good news is most of those opinions are wrong!

Let's separate fact from fiction. Here you'll find only scientific and evidence-based answers to your pregnancy questions and concerns. Some of the answers may surprise you, but much of what you have heard and read about pregnancy is just not true.

What's first?

Hopefully, you are already taking a prenatal vitamin (or at least a folic acid supplement); if you're not, go ahead and start one. You need anything with at least 400 mcg of folic acid in it (per day). You will need more than this if you are on certain medicines for seizures or if you have had a prior pregnancy affected by a neural tube defect. There is no evidence that a different type of folate is better for patients with the MTHFR gene mutation (or that screening for this mutation is beneficial). Next, you should schedule an appointment with your obstetrician or midwife soon. In most cases, there's usually no reason to go in before you are six weeks pregnant. We'll talk about what happens at your prenatal visits in a little bit.

Wait, how far along am I?

Great question. How your due date is calculated is often confusing and different from what you might expect. Pregnancy is 40 weeks, or 280 days, long when measuring from the first day of the last menstrual period. But conception occurs usually two weeks after the first day of the last menstrual period. This means that at the time of conception, a woman is already two weeks pregnant when measured this way. This assumes that her menstrual cycles are 28 days apart.

There are plenty of pregnancy due date apps and calculators that will tell you your estimated due date (EDD) based upon the first day of your last menstrual period (LMP). Calculating your EDD from your LMP assumes a few things:

- That you remember the first day of your last menstrual period correctly.
- That you weren't on birth control or something that would alter your cycles at the time of conception.
- That you have regular, 28-day cycles.

If your cycles are shorter or longer, your due date must be adjusted. If you don't remember when your period was or were on birth control at the time, you will probably have to be dated by an ultrasound. The earlier the ultrasound is performed, the more accurate it is for estimating your due date. Your doctor or midwife will help you figure out an exact due date at your first or second visit.

Many times, women don't remember the exact day of their last menstrual period, or they may not have menstrual cycles that are exactly 28 days long, or they might have been on birth control at the time of conception. Sometimes women ovulate a little bit later than usual, or the bleeding they thought was their last menstrual period was related to the pregnancy (e.g., implantation bleeding). All these factors mean that dating based on the last menstrual period is wrong about 40% of the time. Your doctor or midwife will determine your due date based on your last menstrual period and compare that to a due date determined by the earliest ultrasound, and in some cases, your due date will need to change based on the ultrasound.

As we said, the earliest ultrasound that you have is the best one to determine your due date. Sometimes, patients are confused because subsequent ultrasounds will show measurements that have a slightly different due date, and they will wonder if their due date should be changed again based on these later ultrasounds. The answer is no. The later ultrasounds reflect a pregnancy that is just a little bigger or smaller than the average for that gestational age or vary just because of the margin of error of the scan.

Make sure you clarify at one of your first prenatal visits what your final estimated due date is; then, don't get too fixed on that day. Only

2% of women deliver on their due date. Maybe we should've called it a due month!

But, I don't have a doctor!

If you don't have a doctor yet (or even if you do), you might wonder what you should look for in an OB/GYN. The world is full of advice about this question, but here's ours:

- A good OB will have a low Cesarean delivery rate (don't be afraid to ask - if they don't know their rate, it's probably too high).
- A good OB will ***almost never*** cut episiotomies.
- A good OB will be okay with letting you do almost anything during your pregnancy or delivery.
- A good OB will be supportive of a trial of labor after Cesarean delivery (TOLAC).
- A good OB will not push you towards elective induction of labor.
- A good OB will listen to your concerns and offer evidence-based answers to your questions.

Sometimes the best place to start is by picking the hospital where you would like to deliver. Don't be afraid to call the birth units of your local hospitals and ask these same questions. A lot of hospitals have Cesarean rates well above 30% - even above 50%. Those are probably places to avoid.

If you have specific concerns, ask for specific examples. Let's say you have had a previous Cesarean and want to attempt to have a vaginal birth after Cesarean (VBAC); don't just ask whether a doctor or hospital will allow women to try to have a vaginal birth. Instead, ask them what percentage of their eligible patients attempt a VBAC and how many are successful.

Many providers have learned to say the right things to get patients in the door, but they don't support things like VBAC or external cephalic version (turning a breech baby so that it's head-down to avoid a Cesarean) or vaginal delivery of twin pregnancies. So, ask them how often they do those things if they are relevant to your pregnancy - not just whether they will "let" you try. Don't be afraid to ask questions.

Hopefully, you already have a doctor or midwife that you know and trust or will find one soon. If you are stuck seeing someone who you think isn't quite what you want, don't be afraid to switch. Remember, it's your pregnancy – not theirs.

What happens at my prenatal visits?

Your regular prenatal visits are designed to help maximize your health and the health of your baby, as well as deal with any problems that come up and answer any questions that you might have. The course of your care will vary a bit depending on your individual health and risk factors. In general, here's what to expect at typical prenatal visits.

Confirmation of pregnancy visit

This is usually the first visit you will have, shortly after you find out you are pregnant. Your doctor will confirm you are pregnant and try to establish a final due date, often with an ultrasound. Usually, your doctor will order your prenatal labs and deal with any current or preexisting issues, like medicines you might be taking that need to be stopped or symptoms you may be experiencing.

Your prenatal labs consist of:

- A CBC (complete blood count) to check for anemia and other blood disorders.
- A blood test for syphilis, HIV, hepatitis B, and hepatitis C.
- Your blood type and whether you have any unusual antibodies in your blood that could affect the pregnancy.
- A rubella titer to see if you are immune to rubella.
- A urine drug screen and urine culture. A urine culture should be done ideally before 12 weeks' gestation to identify asymptomatic bacteriuria that might cause problems.

Depending on risk factors, your doctor may add other tests, such as screening for diabetes or sickle cell anemia; and depending on your family history, you may also need screening for genetic diseases like cystic fibrosis or other familial conditions like bleeding or clotting disorders.

We will ask you a series of questions relating to your pregnancy history, medical and surgical history, family history, etc. These detailed series of questions are helpful to screen for any risk factors you may have for your pregnancy.

Some midwives or doctors will order tests at this visit that we usually don't recommend for most patients. These include tests for thyroid function (unless you have a history of thyroid problems or certain symptoms), vitamin D levels, or a blood test for Herpes.

New OB visit

At this visit, we might do a general physical exam of things like your heart. Sometimes you may need a Pap smear and cultures for chlamydia and gonorrhea if these things have not already been done. Not every woman will need a Pap smear (you don't need one *just because* you're pregnant!), so in most cases a pelvic exam may be unnecessary, and we can check for chlamydia and gonorrhea in your urine. Pap smears are generally done no more often than every three years from age 21-30 and every five years after that until age 65.

We also don't recommend a breast or pelvic exam just because you're pregnant. So, chances are, you should be able to keep your clothes on at your first visit. We will review your prenatal lab test results, go over any issues identified from your history, and talk about other pregnancy concerns you may have.

How often will I come for visits?

At the first visit and every visit thereafter, we will check your weight, blood pressure, and, if possible, listen to the fetal heartbeat. This isn't always easy before 12 weeks of pregnancy without an ultrasound. We check your urine at several visits for signs of infection and for protein, which is sometimes associated with the development of preeclampsia if you develop hypertension.

You should always tell us if you are having any symptoms of a urinary tract infection, such as new onset burning with urination or urinary frequency. We will talk about any problems you are having and things you should be looking out for.

Pregnancy is around 40 weeks long (which isn't exactly nine calendar months). We will see you about once a month until 28 weeks, then every two to four weeks until about 36 weeks depending on risk factors, then weekly until you deliver. The exact visit frequency varies and may change as complications or new risk factors develop during your pregnancy.

Sometimes a pelvic exam may be required, particularly if you are bleeding, leaking fluid, or have been having a lot of contractions or other labor symptoms. There's usually not a reason to have your cervix checked at your later visits. These exams don't predict when you might go into labor and are generally unnecessary unless you're having labor symptoms or are planning an induction.

What vaccines do I need during pregnancy?

If you are pregnant during flu season, you should have a **flu shot** as soon as it's available. We also recommend that you stay up to date with any needed **COVID booster shots** which you can receive during pregnancy, if needed. Seasonal flu and COVID infections are a leading cause of maternal death and pregnancy complications, and these vaccines are highly effective and safe. If you are between 32-36 weeks' gestation during the months of September to January, you should also receive the **RSV vaccine** to protect your newborn against RSV infection in those peak months after birth.

We also recommend the **Tdap vaccine** during each pregnancy to protect you and your newborn against whooping cough (pertussis). We recommend this between 27-36 weeks' gestation to optimize the production and transmission of antibodies across the placenta to protect your newborn. If you happen to receive this shot earlier in pregnancy for some reason (maybe you stepped on a nail), you don't need to repeat it later.

What happens at my other visits?

Here are some additional things to know about a few specific visits:

10-12 weeks. Some women may choose to do optional testing for fetal chromosomal abnormalities. Past and current testing strategies focus mostly on Down syndrome (trisomy 21) but as tests have improved, several other conditions can be detected as well. Currently, the preferred way of early screening is called **noninvasive prenatal screening (NIPS)**.

NIPS is a blood test that can be performed any time after 10 weeks' gestation and it screens for Down, Edward (trisomy 18), and Patau (trisomy 13) syndromes, as well as conditions related to an abnormal numbers of sex chromosomes like Turner syndrome (monosomy X); it can also be used to determine the baby's sex. NIPS is now available to all patients who want it (it used to be available only to women with risk factors); it is a much better test than the previously used first trimester screening and detects more abnormalities with far fewer false-positive results.

First trimester screening is a combination of an ultrasound that looks at the thickness of the back of the baby's neck and a blood test for two markers called PAPP-A and HCG. It was previously used to screen for Down syndrome and Edward syndrome. The test also may indicate certain types of heart defects. The test is performed between 11- and 13-weeks' gestation and needs to be ordered in advance. Generally, this test should no longer be performed. Compared to NIPS, there is a high rate of false discoveries and unnecessary anxiety and workups related to those false discoveries. About 5% of patients who take the test will have a positive result; this positive result indicates an actual problem less than 1% of the time, so most positive results are false positives. What's more, about 15% of cases of Down and Edward syndrome are missed by this test.

In contrast, NIPS detects more than 99% of these syndromes and most positive results are true positives. Still, NIPS isn't perfect. In most cases, further testing would be needed to confirm any positive result. This could be done with an **amniocentesis** after 15 weeks' gestation or with **chorionic villus sampling (CVS)** before then. These tests are invasive and carry some risks, so not all patients will choose to have them performed.

16-20 weeks. In this timeframe, usually closer to 20 weeks, all women will receive a detailed **anatomic ultrasound** looking at many specific parts of the fetal anatomy, including all the major organs. This helps to screen for many types of birth defects and other problems.

In the past, women were also offered a test called the **quad screen** during this time. This is a blood test (consisting of four markers: AFP, HCG, Estriol, and Inhibin-A) which screens for Down and Edward syndrome, as well as neural tube defects like spina bifida, abdominal wall defects like gastroschisis, and a few other problems. Like first trimester screening, this test offers no advantages over NIPS and most abnormal results are false discoveries, so it generally should no longer be performed. Some doctors will order a part of this test, the **AFP (alpha fetal protein)**, to screen for neural tube defects. We don't recommend this as it is not evidence-based.

28 weeks. At this visit, all women whose blood type is Rh negative (such as A negative, B negative, O negative, or AB negative) will receive an injection of **Anti-D antibody**, commonly known as **RhoGAM, HyperRHO, BayRHO-D, Rhophylac** or **WinRho.** This injection helps prevent mothers from forming antibodies against their baby's blood, which might be a different blood type from their own.

Between 24- and 28-weeks' gestation, you will have a screening test for **gestational diabetes**. This usually consists of drinking 50 grams of glucose and having your blood sugar checked in an hour. You don't have to be fasting for this test but try not to eat anything big for a couple of hours before. If you fail this test, it doesn't mean that you have gestational diabetes, but it will require you to take a three-hour test. For the three-hour test, you must be fasting. You will drink 100 grams of glucose and your blood sugar will be checked four times: before you consume the drink and at one, two, and three hours. If two or more of these glucose checks are abnormal, then you will be diagnosed with gestational diabetes.

This visit is also a good time to discuss plans for **birth control** after you deliver. If you are planning on having your tubes tied, it is important to let us know at this visit so we can discuss all your options. Also at this visit, depending on risk factors, we may repeat your CBC to check for anemia.

28-32 weeks. It is currently recommended that pregnant women have a repeat test for syphilis during this period even if the first test was negative and regardless of individual risk factors. Depending on your risk factors, other repeat tests may also be performed, such as a CBC or repeat testing for HIV or other tests as indicated by your medical history.

36-37 weeks. Almost every woman will have a swab taken of the vagina, perineum, and anus for **group B Streptococcus (GBS)**. Around one-third of women carry this bacterium as part of their normal genital flora, and it causes no problems for those who do; but it can sometimes cause serious problems for newborns.

If your test is positive, you will need to receive antibiotics in your IV when you are in labor to reduce the risk that your baby will be affected. Ideally, you will get the antibiotic at least four hours before your baby is born. Women with certain risk factors, such as a GBS positive urine culture during pregnancy, or a few other rare situations, won't receive this test and will just be treated empirically during their labors.

You will usually start weekly visits after 36-37 weeks' gestation, and we will begin discussing plans for your delivery.

41 weeks. If you've made it a week past your due date, it's almost always time to be induced. For most women, the risks of continuing the pregnancy are greater than the risks of being induced for both the mother and the newborn.

Other Tests

Depending on your individual circumstances and risk factors, some additional testing may be required for you or your baby. Here are some of the more common ones:

Biophysical profile (BPP). This is an ultrasound test that assesses the well-being of your fetus. It measures the amount of amniotic fluid, the fetal movements, muscle tone, and determines if the fetus is practicing breathing by moving its diaphragm. This may be ordered routinely once per week starting at 32 weeks for women with certain medical problems or complications, and it also may be used intermittently if, for example, the baby is moving less often than normal.

Nonstress test (NST). This test is also used to assess the well-being of your fetus and is used in a similar way as the biophysical profile. In this case, the fetal heart rate is traced for about twenty minutes and then analyzed by the physician. You will be asked to note every time you feel a movement of the baby. The fetal heart rate usually increases (an acceleration) when the baby moves and seeing this is very reassuring. If this happens twice in 20 minutes, we say that the tracing is reactive.

Growth ultrasounds. For some women at increased risk of a very large or a very small baby, we will follow the fetal growth every three to four weeks with an ultrasound. Ultrasound is not a very good way to estimate how big a baby is due to its margin of error (up to 20%), but the trend over time can tell us if there might be a problem. If the growth is small (fetal growth restriction), we may also measure the flow of blood through the umbilical cord to the placenta to check on the health of the placenta (umbilical artery doppler velocimetry).

Amniocentesis. This is a relatively safe procedure where a needle, under ultrasound guidance, is passed through the abdomen into the uterus and some amniotic fluid is collected. This allows us to test many things, including the chromosomes of the fetus if we need to test for something like Down syndrome, for example.

Other lab tests. Some circumstances may arise that require additional lab testing. If, for example, you develop high blood pressure (hypertension), we may check some additional blood work as well as a 24-hour urine collection to look for protein. This is used to test for a serious condition called **preeclampsia**.

If you are having a lot of itching, particularly without a rash, we will check your liver function and check your fasting bile salts. This is used to check for an important condition called **cholestasis of pregnancy.**

If you have any preexisting health problems, you may need certain additional tests to see how well-controlled those conditions are. If you are at high-risk for diabetes or already have it, we will check to see how your blood sugar control is doing. If you have had problems with your thyroid, we will run tests for it. If you have high blood pressure, we will do some tests to see if your major organs, like your kidneys, have been affected by it. There are many other conditions that might require individualized testing.

Do I need to take anything besides my prenatal vitamin?

In most cases, the answer is no. There is a whole industry that markets supplements and other products to pregnant women. Even among prenatal vitamins, for most women the only ingredient that is required is folate, and folate is only necessary until the baby's neural tube is closed, which happens early in the first trimester. The truth is prenatal vitamins are best taken beginning at least two to three months before pregnancy and provide little to no benefit past the first half of the first trimester. In fact, if you are beyond six weeks and prenatal vitamins are making you nauseous or constipated, there's no reason for you to keep taking them.

Aside from the folate in a prenatal vitamin, the other ingredients often found in these vitamins are not evidence-based. Don't get caught up in buying the most expensive prenatal vitamin because the company says it will make your child smarter or reduce the risks of pregnancy; this simply is not true.

In some cases, due to restrictive diets or preexisting anemia or other risk factors, your doctor might ask you to take an additional supplement or medication, most commonly iron.

I'm over 35. What does that mean?

Women who are over 35 years old at the time of delivery receive the label **advanced maternal age (AMA)**. This label was created in the 1970s primarily because of the increasing risk of Down syndrome, which is 1 in 270 at age 35. This cut-off was picked in the 1970s because 1 in 270 was the expected pregnancy loss rate when genetic amniocentesis was performed; at the time invasive testing like amniocentesis was the only choice, and it made sense to only offer it to the highest risk women.

Today, we have noninvasive tests like NIPS available to screen for Down syndrome and we also know that the rate of pregnancy loss with genetic amniocentesis guided by ultrasound is dramatically lower than 1 in 270.

Apart from this increased risk of Down syndrome, being over 35 may not mean much of anything. Typically, as women get older, they may gain extra pounds and extra illnesses that would tend to complicate pregnancies. Yet, a healthy woman of normal body weight above age 35 who does not have a pregnancy complicated by Down syndrome should expect to have a better and safer pregnancy than a woman 10 years her junior who is obese or has a preexisting medical condition. So, your doctor should individualize what your age means for you in the context of your total health status.

We currently recommend some extra antenatal tests for pregnant women over age 40 towards the end of the pregnancy, but between ages 35 and 40, the need for any extra testing should be based upon your individual risk factors and the presence of other medical conditions or illnesses.

Here is the risk of Down syndrome by age and by trimester:

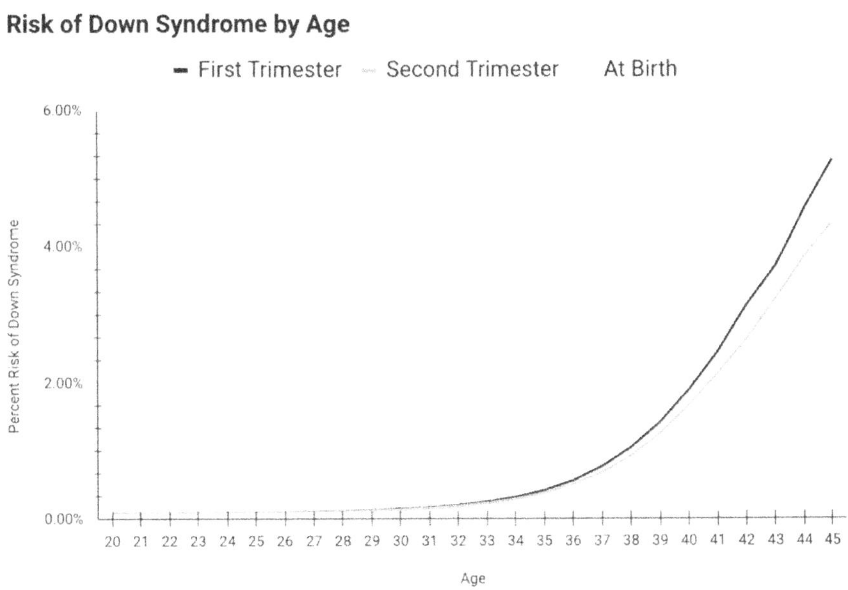

Here is the same risk expressed as one case of Down Syndrome per *X* number of women at *Y* years of age:

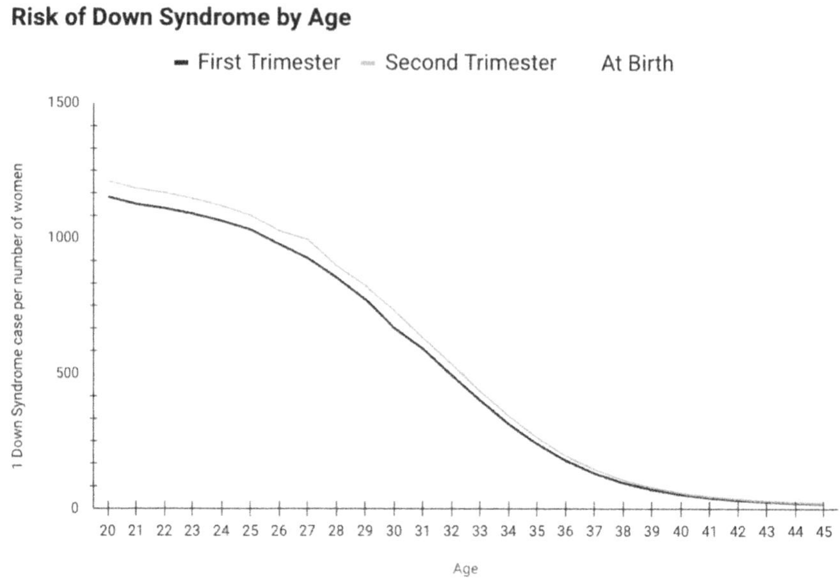

Women today frequently delay childbearing until after age 35 and while this does increase their risk of miscarriage and conditions like Down syndrome, most have pregnancies whose outcomes are like those of younger women. It is also harder to get pregnant the older you get.

Down syndrome is the most common chromosomal abnormality affecting pregnancy, but there are many other chromosomal abnormalities, as well as thousands of genetic and structural abnormalities. Most of these are not detected with routine testing, including ultrasound.

When can I find out the baby's sex?

Most women have traditionally learned the sex of their baby at the time of the anatomy ultrasound, at around 18 to 20 weeks. Today, most women find out earlier. If you happen to have an ultrasound any time after 14 weeks, usually the sex is visible. Ultrasounds at around 12 weeks can sometimes lead to a guess about the fetal sex (the angle of the dangle), but these guesses are only about 85% accurate.

If you choose to have NIPS performed, this includes the fetal sex so you may be able to find out as soon as 11 weeks' gestation if you do the test at 10 weeks' gestation.

Some women choose to not find out the sex of their baby until after it is born, but most women want to know. If you're planning a gender reveal party, make sure you tell your doctor and your sonographer ahead of time, so they don't give away something accidentally. They can always put the answer in a sealed envelope. If you don't want to find out until after the baby is born, make sure you tell whoever might do an ultrasound at any time that you don't want to know; if it's a later ultrasound, they will assume that you already know, and they may say or show something that you don't want to see.

The scientific ways of determining the fetal sex are:

- Ultrasound
- Noninvasive prenatal testing
- Amniocentesis
- Chorionic villus sampling

There are also some not so scientific ways that you'll read about on the Internet. None of these work:

- Chinese gender charts
- Fetal heart rate (under 140=boy, over 140=girl)
- Wedding ring test (pendulum=boy, circle=girl)
- Peeing on Drano (brown=boy, no color change=girl)
- Carrying high vs low (low=boy, high=girl)
- Morning sickness (absent or mild=boy, present or severe=girl)
- Location of weight (belly=boy, hips and butt=girl)
- Placental location (right=boy, left=girl)

Most of these are harmless fun, but there are some products on the market that take advantage of these myths. Don't waste your money.

Dos & Don'ts

How much weight should I gain?

If you started pregnancy at a normal weight, you only burn about 90 additional Calories per day in the first trimester, 275 additional Calories per day in the second trimester, and 500 additional Calories per day in the third trimester.

Normal weight women (BMI of 18.5-24.9) can aim to gain about 25-35 pounds during their pregnancies. Underweight women (BMI < 18.5) may need to gain more and overweight women less. It should be noted that these recommendations are based on averages rather than outcomes data, meaning there is likely a wide range of healthy weight trends that can vary based on individual factors. In general, women who maintain enough hydration and caloric intake to function, and who are not binge eating, will not have pregnancy complications related to weight changes regardless of what their actual trend is. It's a myth that women should "eat for two." Eating can be hard enough as it is when you're pregnant, so eat what you can, don't overeat, and you should be fine. If you have any digestive disorders, you may need additional attention directed towards these conditions, but they are generally very manageable. Most weight gain comes in the second half of pregnancy and often women have gained no weight or even lost weight by their 20th week; this is normal and okay.

If you're pregnant with twins (or more!), the expected weight gain will be a little more than the averages for singleton pregnancies. Expected or average weight gain and optimal weight gain aren't necessarily the same thing. We check your weight at every visit, but please don't focus on how much you gain. While excess weight gain increases the risks of several pregnancy complications, including the risks of preeclampsia, diabetes, fetal macrosomia (a big baby), and

Cesarean delivery, those risks are mainly affected by pre-pregnancy weight rather than how much you gain during pregnancy.

Many overweight women either gain no weight for the entire pregnancy or even lose some weight if they're actively dieting. This is not a bad thing. Maternal weight gain, if it is excessive, is associated with a larger fetal size; but that doesn't mean that gaining very little weight during pregnancy will make your baby too small (if you are overweight at the start of the pregnancy). The goal is to have a healthy baby and a healthy mom. Talk with your doctor or midwife about what your weight journey should look like throughout pregnancy based on your pre-pregnancy weight.

What can't I eat?

This is a great question. The truth is you can eat just about anything you want. Here is the quick and overly cautious answer:

Don't eat:

- Big fish with high levels of mercury, such as shark, swordfish, king mackerel, and tilefish (more than one serving per day)
- Unpasteurized milk and soft cheeses
- Raw or undercooked meats
- Cold cuts (lunch meat, salami, etc.)

Here are the explanations:

Because of high levels of **mercury** in some big fish, pregnant women should avoid shark, swordfish, king mackerel, and tilefish. Smaller fish are usually safe, such as light tuna, salmon, pollock, and catfish. Up to 12 ounces per week of these fish is considered safe. In fact, regular consumption of fish (and their omega fats) has been associated with lower rates of preterm labor and other complications of pregnancy. Recent evidence suggests that even the recommendation about avoiding the larger fish is likely unnecessary. So don't stress too much unless you happen to eat these larger fish in multiple meals a day, multiples times per week.

Listeriosis is a rare type of food poisoning that can affect pregnant women and cause stillbirths. To avoid this, you should wash all fruits and vegetables before eating them and avoid eating unpasteurized milk or soft cheeses, raw or undercooked meats, poultry, or shellfish. Ideally, hot dogs and deli meats should be heated thoroughly prior to eating though the absolute risk of acquiring listeria from deli meats is extraordinarily low. Don't be too freaked out about listeria; most women take a greater chance just by driving to the doctor's office than by eating high-risk foods. The absolute risk of anything happening from eating any of these foods is incredibly low. While you shouldn't worry too much, pregnancy isn't the time to explore strange and new foods from uncertain sources.

What can I do?

It's amazing how many things you'll hear you shouldn't do while pregnant. Family members and perfect strangers are all happy to offer advice. But remember, most of that advice may be wrong. Unfortunately, any time something bad happens in pregnancy, like a miscarriage or preterm delivery, patients (and doctors) tend to blame whatever happened *just before* that bad thing; this type of anecdotal evidence gets passed on to others. But scientific research simply doesn't support most of these claims. Let's look at some common things.

Can I drink caffeine?

Yes, you can. As with most things in life, moderation is the key. Scientific studies have not demonstrated any problems with caffeine consumption during pregnancy until a woman consumes over 700 mg per day. That's a lot of caffeine! To be safe, and to make sure that a woman never approaches that amount of caffeine consumption, we recommend that pregnant women limit themselves to 350 mg of caffeine per day.

In general, you are okay to keep your morning routine if it consists of an average cup of regular coffee or the average serving of a caffeinated soft drink. But beware, it is possible to overdo it with a large special order from Starbucks. If you drink a lot of caffeine prior to pregnancy, cutting it out altogether can produce daily headaches. All things in moderation, including caffeine.

Most soft drinks have about 40 mg per 12 ounces (Diet Coke has 46 mg). Most coffee has around 75 mg per eight ounces, but this amount varies widely. Most teas have around 40 mg per eight ounces, and energy drinks like Red Bull have about 80 mg per can.

Check out this website at the QR code for the amount of caffeine in your favorite beverage.

Can I exercise while I'm pregnant?

Yes. The short answer is that exercise is a beneficial activity throughout pregnancy and virtually all pregnant women should exercise. Almost every limitation to exercise that you have heard or read elsewhere on the Internet is not evidence-based. Women who exercise have better pregnancies in every aspect. Let's talk more about exercise briefly.

Exercise is not only healthy during pregnancy, but it improves pregnancy outcomes! Pregnant women who exercise have less backaches, bloating, constipation, swelling, and gestational diabetes. They have improved energy, mood, posture, and sleep. Some studies have even shown that exercise can prevent gestational diabetes and increase the chance of having a vaginal delivery.

Historically, it was falsely assumed that physical activity could increase the risk of miscarriage, preterm deliveries, or contribute to growth restriction of the fetus. There have been drastic shifts in evidence pointing away from these concerns. There is no longer a restriction of maximum heart rate (no different from a non-pregnant woman, anyway). Healthy women should get at least 150 minutes (2 hours and 30 minutes, at least 10 minutes at a time) per week of moderate-intensity aerobic activity (such as brisk walking) during and after their pregnancy.

Healthy women who already do a vigorous-intensity aerobic activity (such as running) or large amounts of other vigorous activity can continue doing so during and after their pregnancy. For women that want to begin physical activity during pregnancy, the activity should be gradually increased over time, working up to the moderate intensity recommendations described above.

Pilates and yoga for pregnancy help with strength and flexibility. Walking, swimming, cycling, aerobics, and running are all safe and provide good cardiovascular exercise during pregnancy. Studies have shown that blood flow to the baby improves during cardiovascular exercise. It makes sense to not over-exert yourself to the point of being short of breath, but vigorous cardiovascular exercise (and even weightlifting, within reason) is safe during pregnancy and you don't need to worry about how fast your heart rate is.

Here are some examples of moderate-intensity activities:

- Walking
- Hiking
- Bicycling at 5 to 9 mph
- Aerobic dancing
- Water aerobics
- Dancing
- Doubles tennis
- Golf
- Recreational swimming
- Gardening
- Housework
- Playing with children or pets

And here are some examples of vigorous-intensity activities:

- Jogging or running
- Backpacking
- Bicycling more than 10 mph or on a hilly terrain
- Step aerobics
- Fast-paced dancing
- Singles tennis
- Soccer
- Swimming laps
- Shoveling snow
- Moving furniture
- Vigorously playing with children or running with pets

Signs or symptoms that you should stop exercising include vaginal bleeding, feeling faint, chest pain, headache, calf pain or swelling, uterine contractions, or fluid leaking from the vagina.

Obviously, avoid contact sports during pregnancy as well as other activities in which there is a high risk of falling (e.g., gymnastics, horseback riding, water skiing, etc.). Also, avoid downhill skiing and SCUBA diving.

There are some medical or pregnancy conditions where exercise or certain types of exercise might need to be limited. Some examples include:

- Significant heart disease
- Restrictive lung disease
- Placenta previa in the third trimester
- Short cervical length diagnosed in the second trimester

- Persistent second or third trimester vaginal bleeding
- Premature labor
- Ruptured membranes (broken water)
- Preeclampsia

If you are unsure if you have any of these conditions, talk to your obstetrician or midwife about your medical history.

Unfortunately, as of 2011, 85% of pregnant women did not meet the recommended guidelines for exercise during pregnancy. Don't be one of the 85%!

Is it okay to have sex during pregnancy?

Yes! There are some rare reasons for a woman to abstain from sex during pregnancy. These rare cases where the risks may outweigh the benefits include certain cases of preterm labor with advanced cervical dilation; preterm, premature rupture of membranes; or placenta or vasa previa. Also, women who have had a cervical cerclage during pregnancy should probably abstain, though the evidence is uncertain. Otherwise, have fun!

Most women find sex during pregnancy more satisfying and pleasurable than outside of pregnancy. Sex during pregnancy is not associated with an increased risk of miscarriage, preterm labor, or any other complications of pregnancy. Even in cases where penetration may not be the best idea, such as the situations listed above, orgasms during pregnancy are still perfectly fine. If you have a cervical cerclage and don't need penetration to orgasm, then feel free to enjoy yourself!

As your uterus gets bigger during pregnancy, different sexual positions may help both with comfort and satisfaction. If you are having trouble with comfort during sex, ask your doctor about it.

Can I go to the dentist?

Yes – please do. Good dental hygiene is associated with good pregnancy outcomes. A severely infected tooth, on the other hand, may lead to problems for the pregnancy. There are no routine practices at the dentist's office that are unsafe during pregnancy. This includes pulling teeth and getting dental x-rays. A pregnant woman can undergo many tens of thousands of shielded dental x-rays during pregnancy without fear of delivering a harmful amount of radiation exposure to the pregnancy.

Local anesthetics, antibiotics, and pain medicines that are commonly used by dentists are all also safe during pregnancy. If your dentist has a question about a particular antibiotic or other medicine, have them ask your obstetrician.

Can I get a massage while I'm pregnant?

Yes. It is a myth, sometimes perpetuated by massage therapists themselves, that massages can be so relaxing they might stimulate preterm labor. This is false. Some massage therapists may want a note from your doctor stating that a massage is safe, and we can't think of a good reason why your doctor wouldn't give you such a note, if needed.

Can I dye my hair while I'm pregnant?

Yes! The Internet is full of advice recommending that you don't dye your hair while pregnant, at least in the first trimester. This is born out of ignorance and a fear of everything during the first trimester. There is no scientific data which says that dying your hair is associated with any adverse problems, even in the first trimester. If you think about it, most female beauticians and hair stylists also become pregnant at some time, and they are exposed to these chemicals hundreds or thousands of times more than what you are exposed to when getting your hair dyed. We don't recommend that women change their occupation while pregnant.

Should I wear my seatbelt while I'm pregnant?

Yes! The best way to protect your baby during pregnancy is to protect yourself. Seatbelts are the best way to do this while driving. It is a myth that seat belts add extra or unnecessary risks to your baby; on the contrary, they may save your life and your baby's life. Buckle up!

Can I travel while I'm pregnant?

In general, the answer is yes. Under normal circumstances, travel during pregnancy is safe until the last 5 weeks or so of pregnancy. This includes flying. Most cruise ships will not allow you embark if you are pregnant past a certain gestational age. Be sure to drink plenty of fluids, walk, and stretch your legs on long trips.

You should take normal precautions while traveling, such as wearing seat belts. The lap belt should be below your belly so that it fits snugly across your hips and pelvic bone; the shoulder belt should be across your chest (between your breasts) and over the mid-portion of your collarbone (away from your neck). Never place the shoulder belt under your arm or behind your back. Ensure there is no slack in the belt and that your airbags are turned to "on." Keep 10 inches between the steering wheel and your breastbone. You may need to angle the steering wheel toward your breasts, not your belly or head.

There is nothing inherently dangerous about traveling by ground, sea, or plane during pregnancy. However, you do have to consider how long you will be separated from the ability to seek medical care and how far away that medical care might be. This is more important in the third trimester, particularly in the late third trimester when labor is more likely. It's for this reason that many cruise ships will not allow you to embark after 24 weeks' gestation. They do not want any liability related to premature delivery when the baby has a chance to survive preterm. It's not that sailing isn't safe – only that it can take you many hours away from a hospital.

Planes do not often limit travel by gestational age, but you should consider how long your flight is. There is a big difference between flying from Atlanta to New York versus flying from New York to Melbourne. In general, many doctors recommend avoiding flying after 35 weeks' if the length of the flight is particularly long.

Some people worry about traveling by car due to the concern of an increased risk of blood clots secondary to the immobilization of sitting in a car. This is probably not a valid reason to avoid travel by car, particularly when you consider that pregnant women will be taking pit stops every two or three hours anyway. When you stop for a bathroom break, be sure to walk around for a couple of minutes.

Does it matter how I sleep?

A lot of women ask this question because they've been told to never sleep on their back, particularly in the third trimester. Most advice on the Internet and in books about pregnancy recommends against sleeping on your back. There is no good scientific evidence that sleeping on the back increases the risk of stillbirth or other problems, even in the third trimester. There have been studies that show that fetuses have some fetal heart rate changes while the mother is sleeping on her back, but these changes have not been definitively associated with an increased risk of stillbirth. Studies of observed sleeping habits show that women roll around a lot and likely have little control over how they lie while they are asleep.

Women in the third trimester are unlikely to sleep on their backs naturally due to their belly size, so they tend to sleep on one side or the other anyway. If they do sleep on their backs, there is little to do about it since women have no control over how they turn and roll during sleep. Since there has been no definitive connection between back sleeping and stillbirth, women should not lose too much sleep (pun intended) worrying about how they sleep.

Pregnancy Q&A

What medications should I stop?

Because researchers don't conduct drug safety experiments on pregnant patients, we can never guarantee the safety of any medicine in pregnancy. For the most part, we advise avoiding any medications that may be unnecessary, even more so in the first trimester when the fetus is still developing new tissues and organs.

However, many medications are used commonly during pregnancy and are not thought to pose any problems; and many more medicines may have some risks but are necessary to treat serious medical problems that pose even bigger risks if left untreated. The truth is, there are only a few medications that we know you should definitively avoid during pregnancy. These include:

- **ACE-inhibitors** or **angiotensin receptor blockers (ARBs)** such as lisinopril, enalapril, ramipril, captopril, benazepril, irbesartan (Avapro), losartan (Cozaar), olmesartan (Benicar), and valsartan (Diovan). These medications don't cause harm in the first trimester but should be stopped when you become pregnant. Talk to your doctor about a blood pressure medicine that would be safe for you.
- Some **seizure medications**, such as carbamazepine, phenytoin, and valproic acid. There are safer alternatives to treat seizure disorders and your doctor can help you transition to a safer medicine.
- **Lithium.** This medicine is used to treat bipolar disorder and can usually be replaced with a safer medication.
- Some **antibiotics** including streptomycin, kanamycin, tetracycline, and fluoroquinolones, such as ciprofloxacin or levofloxacin, should not be used.
- The blood thinner **warfarin** should almost always be avoided.

- The relatively new weight loss and diabetes medications, including **semaglutide** (Ozempic), **tirzepatide** (Mounjaro, Zepbound), and others, have been minimally studied in pregnant patients. Animal studies have shown possible harm. We recommend avoiding these drugs while actively trying to get pregnant and certainly after pregnancy is confirmed.
- **Methotrexate.** This medicine is used for many things, including rheumatoid arthritis, but should not be used in pregnancy.

There are many, many other medications that should be avoided during pregnancy and you should ask your doctor about your medicines and supplements at your first visit.

What over-the-counter medicines can I use?

Most over-the-counter medications are safe to use for common pregnancy complaints. Here are some common medicines and remedies that you should feel comfortable using for different problems:

- **Headaches:** Tylenol (acetaminophen). NSAID medications like Motrin or Aleve should be avoided in the third trimester but are safe to take through the second trimester.
- **Nausea:** vitamin B6 (at least 25 mg two times per day); Unisom SleepTabs (doxylamine) (half a tablet during the day or a whole tablet at night), Benadryl (diphenhydramine).
- **Heartburn:** Mylanta, Maalox, TUMS, Rolaids, and other drugs such as Zantac or Pepcid.
- **Diarrhea:** Kaopectate or Imodium (don't treat for the first 24-48 hours).
- **Constipation:** MiraLAX, milk of magnesia, Fibercon, Metamucil, Citrucel.
- **Leg cramps:** oral hydration, calcium supplements.
- **Cold symptoms:** Tylenol.
- **Nasal congestion:** humidifiers, saline drops, Sudafed (if you don't have high blood pressure), Afrin nasal spray, Benadryl. Note that phenylephrine does not work to reduce congestion - it is completely useless and not worth taking during or outside of pregnancy.
- **Sore throat:** Cepacol or similar products, lozenges, etc.
- **Vaginal yeast infection:** Monistat 3 or 7.

- **Gas:** Gas-X, Mylicon
- **Insect bites, rashes:** Benadryl cream, Calamine.
- **Insomnia** or **difficulty falling sleeping:** Unisom SleepTabs, Benadryl, Tylenol PM

Should I be worried about infections?

Cytomegalovirus (CMV) is a virus related to the herpes viruses. It is so common that up to 85% of adults in the United States have been infected at some point in their lives.

Usually, CMV is a mild disease that does not cause any serious problems in healthy children and adults. Most people get flu-like symptoms or cold-like symptoms for a few days, if they develop any symptoms at all. However, some people, including immunocompromised women and newborn babies of women infected with CMV during pregnancy, can have serious complications and even death.

Pregnant women infected with CMV for the first time during pregnancy can pass the virus to their unborn babies. The virus can also pass from mother to baby in vaginal secretions during delivery and in breast milk after birth. The virus can pass from person to person through blood, saliva, breast milk, and urine.

Up to 40% of babies born to women who are newly infected with CMV during pregnancy will become infected. Not all infected babies will have symptoms at birth.

Newborns with CMV are likely to be born early and weigh less. Other possible problems include a small brain (microcephaly) or other nervous system disorders that can cause seizures, deafness, mental retardation, or death. This infection can cause the liver and spleen to become larger than normal, as well as jaundice and blood disorders. Newborns with CMV may have a rash that consists of small bruises called petechiae and larger bruises known as purpura. Some of these findings can be detected prior to birth with ultrasound, but most cannot.

A baby born to a mother who was already infected with CMV *before* she became pregnant is less likely to be born with CMV due to mom's preexisting immunity. Only 0.5% to 1.5% of such babies are infected (compared to 40% of babies born to mothers who were infected for the first-time during pregnancy), and their problems tend to be less severe. There are currently no treatments for maternal or fetal CMV infection.

The pediatrician may order blood tests for babies with low birth weight, jaundice, small brains, or other problems that can be associated with congenital CMV. The diagnosis needs to be confirmed by testing blood or tissue from the infant within three weeks of birth to be accurate.

Young, healthy pregnant women usually do not need to be tested because they do not need to be treated specifically for CMV. They usually recover over a period of weeks. In some instances, blood tests may be done to confirm the cause of the illness, since similar symptoms can be caused by the Epstein-Barr virus (EBV) and even human immunodeficiency virus (HIV). Some of the antibody tests used to test for CMV have a high false-positive rate and the testing needs to be repeated to be reliable.

Pregnant women who care for young children should take these precautions to reduce the risk of CMV:

- Wash hands often with soap and water, especially after changing diapers. Wash well for 15 to 20 seconds.
- Do not kiss young children under the age of five or six on the mouth or cheek. Instead, kiss them on the head or give them a big hug.
- Do not share food, drinks, or utensils (spoons, forks, or knives) with young children.

If you are pregnant and work in a daycare center, reduce your risk of getting CMV by working with children who are older than two and a half years of age, especially if you have never been infected with CMV or are unsure if you have been exposed.

Why am I so tired?

Pregnant women are often excessively tired in the first and third trimesters, but probably for different reasons. In the first trimester, your body undergoes rapid physiological changes accompanied by high levels of hormones that conspire to exhaust you. Couple this with food aversion or nausea and vomiting, and the result for many women is complete exhaustion.

This tends to get better by the second trimester and then in the third trimester, particularly the last few weeks of pregnancy, exhaustion returns as you sleep less at night and carry around 30+ extra pounds during the day. If you have another small baby or two at home already, then the effect is even worse.

To help with symptoms in the first trimester, you can work on minimizing the effects of nausea and vomiting of pregnancy by eating several small meals or snacks throughout the day and adding vitamin B6 twice a day if you haven't already. Naps sometimes feel like a good idea, but they often have the opposite effect than what you desire. Napping can interfere with your ability to get good rest at night, and this can create a vicious cycle. Going for a walk or getting some exercise is probably a better idea and will improve your nighttime sleep.

Some women in the first trimester are excessively tired because they have cut caffeine completely out of their diets. Remember, you can still have up to 350 mg of caffeine per day; so, don't feel too bad about having that cup of coffee in the morning or maybe after lunch.

Many pregnant women need to work on maximizing their sleep hygiene. Make sure you have a dark room, maybe with a noisemaker, like a fan or a white noise generator (there are free apps for your smartphone) to minimize interruptions. Try to use your bedroom for sleep only; don't make a habit of watching TV from your bed or staring at your phone. Pregnant women often find every little uncomfortable spring in their mattresses with their rounder bellies and hips. Try adding an extra layer of egg crate or a foam topper to your mattress and make sure you have a long pillow that you can hug with your legs. A hot shower about an hour before you go to sleep can also make a huge difference.

Be sure to empty your bladder right before you go to sleep and, if you find that you are waking up to pee several times a night, you might need to restrict water intake for a couple of hours before going to sleep. In rare cases, excess fatigue might indicate another problem such as a thyroid abnormality or anemia. If you feel like you are more tired than the average pregnant woman, be sure to talk to your doctor.

If you are occasionally tired or having a difficult time getting to sleep or are tossing and turning, an antihistamine like Unisom SleepTabs or Benadryl can be a safe option to help with sleep. We recommend trying healthy sleeping habits before resorting to medications.

Finally, if you are snoring a lot, you might have sleep apnea. A sleep study and treatment for this can be life-changing! Don't hesitate to talk to your doctor about a sleep study while you're pregnant.

I'm throwing up! Help!

Nausea and vomiting during pregnancy are no one's idea of a good time. Unfortunately, it affects about two-thirds of pregnant women. The good news is, nausea and vomiting are not associated with risks to the pregnancy; the bad news is, you are nauseated and throwing up. What can you do?

- Eat several small meals per day and avoid high-fat foods.
- Eat bland foods and avoid smells that are noxious.
- Increase the protein and liquid content of your food.
- Ginger capsules can help (three 250 mg capsules a day and one before bed).
- Taking a vitamin B6 supplement (25 mg) 2-3 times per day alone or in combination with Unisom SleepTabs (doxylamine) at night may be beneficial.

Your doctor may need to prescribe an anti-nausea medicine for you if these remedies don't resolve the issue. There are several drugs that are safe in pregnancy to choose from, including ondansetron (Zofran), metoclopramide (Reglan), promethazine, haloperidol, and a few others.

Make sure that your acid reflux and constipation are treated since both of those can contribute to nausea and vomiting as well.

In bad cases, you may need to be hospitalized for IV fluids and other treatments if you are unable to keep anything down and experiencing signs of severe dehydration/malnutrition.

Hopefully, you will feel better by the end of the first trimester. If you don't, or if the above remedies are not working, your doctor may need to investigate other causes of your nausea and vomiting apart from pregnancy. Typically, you shouldn't be concerned as long as you can maintain your body weight and stay hydrated during the first trimester. If you lose a few pounds from the nausea and vomiting, it isn't too concerning; but more significant losses should be investigated further.

Is it okay if I don't have morning sickness?

Yes! Count your blessings and don't tell any of your pregnant friends or they'll be very jealous. Some women never get morning sickness and that is completely okay. If you're losing sleep over it, you can always come in to hear the fetal heartbeat.

Is it normal that I'm cramping?

Almost all women have some cramping or other pains during pregnancy, particularly in the first trimester. This cramping is almost never anything to be worried about, especially if you're not bleeding. In the first trimester, the uterus grows rapidly and most of the cramping that a woman experiences is simply growing pains. As the uterus gets bigger, it becomes top-heavy and tends to pull and tug from one side to the other. This will stretch ligaments, particularly the round ligaments of the uterus, and cause either cramping or sharp pains in the groin. None of these symptoms put the baby at risk.

Sometimes cramping is not related to your uterus at all. Many women become constipated during pregnancy and the cramping they experience is related to their bowels slowing down. Sometimes cramping is related to the bladder and might be a sign of bladder infection, but almost always there will be other symptoms like burning when you pee.

In the second and third trimesters, cramping is often what is called Braxton-Hicks contractions. We will talk about these contractions and compare them to real labor contractions later when we answer the question, "How can I tell if I'm in labor?"

Is bleeding any amount normal?

Some amount of bleeding during the first trimester is very common, affecting about one-third of pregnant women. Avoid sex if you are bleeding until you can discuss the bleeding with your doctor and she clears you for normal activities, or it resolves. Bleeding increases your risk of miscarriage, but, surprisingly, not by very much.

If you are having heavy bleeding and cramping, you need to be seen. Bleeding later in pregnancy may be a sign of labor or other problems, but it can also be normal. A lot of women will spot later in pregnancy, especially if their cervix is starting to slowly dilate. Always discuss heavy bleeding with your doctor immediately. This is almost never a reason to go the emergency department, but it is a reason to be seen in the office in the next day or two.

What can I do about constipation?

Constipation is incredibly common during pregnancy. In the 19th century, many called pregnancy the "Disease of Constipation." The good news is that all the remedies and treatments you might normally use for constipation are still safe during pregnancy. If you're struggling with constipation, start by increasing your water and fiber intake. Many women will add daily use of MiraLAX or a generic equivalent to their diet. This is a gentle agent that is non-stimulating and safe to use during pregnancy. If it has been a few days since your last bowel movement, you may need to stimulate a bowel movement from below. Try using a suppository (e.g., glycerin or Dulcolax), and if this doesn't work you can repeat it in two hours.

If these over-the-counter remedies are not helpful, talk to your doctor.

These hemorrhoids are a pain in my ***!

Nobody likes a hemorrhoid. Hemorrhoids don't even like hemorrhoids. Unfortunately, they are common during pregnancy and become more common in the third trimester. All the normal over-the-counter remedies for hemorrhoids are perfectly fine to use while pregnant, including creams like Preparation H and Anusol-HC. Tucks pads, which are pads infused with witch hazel, are also effective. Many women will use the pads in combination with one of the creams.

Most hemorrhoids get significantly better after delivery, though they may get worse with pushing. Sitz baths with added witch hazel may be your best friend in the postpartum period.

Rarely, hemorrhoids become thrombosed and may need to be incised to remove the clot. You should suspect that a hemorrhoid has become thrombosed if you have new, different severe pain that prevents you from being able to sit down. If you're worried about this, ask your doctor immediately.

Heartburn! Help!

You've probably heard the folktale that a lot of heartburn means that your baby will have a lot of hair; this isn't true, and dreams of a well-coiffed baby undoubtedly won't make your pain any better.

Heartburn aka acid reflux aka GERD is a common problem during pregnancy and gets worse throughout the third trimester for most women as the uterus grows and puts more pressure on the stomach. If you have occasional symptoms, avoiding trigger foods and using TUMS may be enough. For persistent symptoms, it is okay to use over-the-counter medications like TUMS, Gaviscon, Maalox, or Mylanta, as well as antacid medications such as proton pump inhibitors (omeprazole, pantoprazole) and antihistamines (cimetidine).

Why am I itching?

Most itching in pregnancy is related to dry skin. A good lotion can go a long way in reducing or eliminating itching related to this problem. In some cases, itching confined to one area may be related to a reaction to something; we call this **contact dermatitis**. If you suspect this is the case, try to avoid whatever you encountered and think about any new lotions, detergents, or other things coming into contact with your skin or clothing. Consider using an antihistamine or an over-the-counter steroid cream to help.

In rare cases, itching all over the body that is not associated with a rash can be due to **intrahepatic cholestasis of pregnancy (ICP)**. ICP is an important diagnosis to not miss, and your doctor may need to check some labs to make sure you don't have this. If you do, she will prescribe medicine to improve the situation and will likely deliver you a couple of weeks earlier than normal.

Lastly, if you have little red dots, plaques, or raised bumps that develop and are itchy during pregnancy, you may have **polymorphic eruption of pregnancy (PEP)**. It most commonly shows up on the belly or legs. We treat this similarly to other rashes with topical steroid creams, antihistamines, or oral steroids if necessary, and soothing baths/lotions/loose clothing can help with the itchiness. When the itching gets bad, trying cold ice packs to calm it down can be very helpful.

When should I feel the baby moving?

If you are less than 20 weeks' gestation or so, you are probably too early to feel any fetal movement. First time moms don't typically report feeling movements for the first time (quickening) until 20 weeks or so. Women who have had children before often feel the first movements two or three weeks sooner (around 17-20 weeks). Even after these gestational ages, it is still common to not feel daily movement until about 24 weeks or so.

After 24 weeks, you should expect to feel some movement every day, but how much movement you feel varies from pregnancy to pregnancy. You or your partner may not be able to feel the baby with a hand on the outside of your belly simply because you have an anterior placenta, or the baby is turned and kicking in the other direction. Once you have started feeling kicks consistently, you should be feeling something at least daily. However, due to the small size of the baby in the second trimester, the frequency and strength of the movements you feel may not be consistent.

If you are concerned that you have not felt enough fetal movement and you are more than 28 weeks' gestation, then lie down on your left side and concentrate on feeling for movements. You should feel at least 6 movements of some sort in the first hour; if you have felt some movements but not 6, continue counting for another hour. You should feel at least 10 movements during those two hours. Because of fetal sleep cycles, it's not uncommon for it to take two hours to feel the 10 movements. Ideally, this is done during the baby's active time. For many women, the baby's active time is shortly after they have eaten dinner. So, maybe try eating a little something if you don't reach the 6 kicks in an hour, and then extend to counting for the two-hour mark. If you don't reach 10 movements in two hours, then this is a reason to go to the hospital or office and be evaluated.

You might have read on the Internet that you should do "kick counts" every day. Most pregnant women do not need to do this as the practice may be harmful overall to the pregnancy. Only do daily kick counts if your doctor has told you to do it for a specific reason.

Can I prevent stretch marks?

The short answer is no. Though there are a lot of products marketed to pregnant women who are willing to spend a lot of money to prevent stretch marks, none of them have good scientific data showing they work. Some products cite their own small studies, but they are usually poorly done or so small that it cannot be considered good evidence. Companies like to exploit new moms, so be leery. We don't want that for you, and you're better off saving your money. If your belly is dry and it feels good to use a nice lotion or other skincare product, go for it! But know that it will not prevent stretch marks. We promise the second we see something come out that is effective and has good data behind it, we'll be the first to tell everyone.

Why are my legs and hands so swollen?

Ah, the joys of pregnancy! If constipation, hemorrhoids, and heartburn weren't enough to make you feel glorious, just wait until your legs start swelling.

Most swelling or edema in pregnancy is normal. Swelling is common; about 60% of women will have significant lower extremity swelling and many these women will also have swelling in their hands that makes rings too tight and wrists hurt. Much of the conventional wisdom about swelling during pregnancy is related to a concern for the development of preeclampsia, but swelling is so common that in most cases this is not a concern at all. Your doctor checks your blood pressure at your regular visits to make sure that you're not developing hypertension, which is the chief sign of preeclampsia.

Most leg swelling is related to the uterus blocking the return of blood from your legs. As the uterus gets bigger, it blocks the veins that drain blood from the legs back up to the heart, and gravity doesn't help with this process. Since the veins in your legs have no muscles or pumps, the blood tends to pool in your legs, and this leads to swelling. You may be able to make this temporarily better by elevating your legs, particularly while laying on your side. But for most women who are up and active throughout the day, there is little opportunity for this. Wearing a pair of support hose, compression stockings, or compression socks may help tremendously. Sleeping or laying down on your left side can also provide an opportunity for blood to drain from your legs.

If your hands are swelling, you may have symptoms of carpal tunnel syndrome which is also very common during pregnancy. Wearing an over-the-counter wrist splint at night on one or both wrists may lead to significant improvement of these painful symptoms.

One common myth about swelling is that a woman should drink more water when she is swelling to make the swelling better. This is simply untrue. If you're having significant swelling in your legs, you may also find that you are lightheaded or having woozy episodes because your water content has left your blood vessels and gone into your soft tissues; in this case, drinking more water may help you not feel as dizzy, but it will not affect how swollen you are.

My back is killing me. What can I do?

Back pain in pregnancy is almost universal. The bigger the belly, the more curved the spine, and the worse the back pain. As your center of gravity moves forward with your ever-increasing belly size, your hips rotate forward, the curvature of your back is altered, and the muscle groups you use to maintain your posture change. Because you are not used to using these muscle groups to stay upright, and because all your muscles are doing more work than normal carrying around the extra weight, the result is chronic muscle strain, sprain, and fatigue.

Things to try include using acetaminophen to treat the pain and if you are less than 28 weeks' gestation, you can still use nonsteroidal anti-inflammatories (NSAIDs) like ibuprofen or Naprosyn occasionally. A heating pad on the back, heat-releasing patches, or a nice bath may also help a lot.

Exercise can help tremendously. Gymnasts and ballet dancers rarely complain of back pain during pregnancy because they have well-developed back musculature and core abdominal muscles. Exercises that help strengthen the back and core abdominal muscles can provide relief and prevent worsening problems as the pregnancy goes on. This includes things like Pilates or Yoga.

Many women benefit from wearing a back brace or pregnancy support belt (belly band). These devices tend to change your center of gravity slightly and help redistribute the load. Typically, these are most helpful in the third trimester. Even if you did not need one in your first pregnancy, keep in mind that during your second or third pregnancy you carry the baby differently in your pelvis and it may be helpful this time around.

Massage can be beneficial, and some women may need help from a physical therapist. Your doctor can let you know if physical therapy or, in some cases, pelvic floor physical therapy, might be appropriate for your symptoms. In some cases, we may prescribe muscle relaxants, but these tend to be sedating. Still, they can be useful at night.

It's unusual for back pain during pregnancy to require any testing or other treatments. However, if you have a history of chronic back pain or orthopedic abnormalities, be sure to tell your doctor or midwife. Various pains, particularly back pain, pelvic pain, and round ligament pain are common in pregnancy.

Here is a list of things that can help relieve pains:

- Stretching and strengthening exercises like Pilates or Yoga
- Wear a pregnancy support belt
- Use Tylenol
- Use warm compresses or pads
- Wear low-heeled shoes with good arch support
- Avoid lifting heavy items by yourself
- Elevate one foot on a support if you must stand for a long period of time

- Bend with your knees, not at the waist
- Try to sleep on your side with one or two pillows between your knees
- Place a board under your mattress to make your bed firmer.

Why can't I breathe?

Nearly 97% of pregnant women complain of shortness of breath at some time during their pregnancies. Most of the time, this is related to some of the pulmonary physiologic changes of pregnancy that give women the sensation that they are not breathing in deeply or moving as much air with each inspiration, but their actual oxygen status remains unchanged. It is normal to feel as if you are not breathing as deeply or have your rate of respirations increase with less vigorous activity while pregnant.

Rarely, difficulty breathing is a sign of a more serious problem. If you're having trouble catching your breath even while resting or if you have symptoms of low oxygen levels, like changes in the color of your skin or confusion, then you may need to seek medical care immediately. Women who have underlying asthma may also have shortness of breath related to uncontrolled asthma during pregnancy and this would be a reason to seek immediate medical attention as well. Also, if you notice that you can't sleep without propping your head up with several pillows, you need to talk to your doctor.

Otherwise, if your shortness of breath is just with exertion and improves with rest, it is likely normal.

What can I do for seasonal allergies?

Brand name or generic versions of Allegra, Zyrtec, or Claritin are safe, but avoid those drugs with the "-D" component because it can elevate your blood pressure. Most other over-the-counter allergy remedies are safe as well.

What can I do for my headache?

Pregnancy can be both good and bad for headaches. The good news is that migraine headaches are uncommon during pregnancy. Most chronic migraineurs thoroughly enjoy pregnancy because it is one of the few times in their lives when they don't suffer from migraine headaches.

The bad news is, other types of headaches, particularly tension headaches, can become more common during pregnancy with the musculoskeletal strains, tensions, anxieties, and stresses associated with pregnancy.

You can always use acetaminophen at any time during pregnancy for headache. If you're less than 28 weeks' gestation, you can still use ibuprofen or Naprosyn. Other medications like Excedrin Migraine can also be used on a limited basis. A good massage, a relaxing bath, or just a good night's rest may be the cure for a tension headache.

Sometimes headaches have other causes, like sinus infections or allergies. If you suspect that your sinuses are the problem, try an over-the-counter antihistamine and if this doesn't work, talk to your doctor.

Some women have caffeine withdrawal headaches, especially in the first trimester. These headaches are all too common if you have recently cut out all caffeine because you're pregnant. Remember that you can have up to 350 mg of caffeine per day. You may need to add a little bit of caffeine back to prevent headaches. Caffeine is also a treatment for some tension headaches as well. Taking your acetaminophen with a serving of caffeine may be just what the doctor ordered.

Why does sex hurt?

Sex is safe during pregnancy and often a lot of fun. Most couples enjoy the body's changes during pregnancy, but sometimes women can find sex painful and problematic.

Some women find it difficult to relax because they're worried that sex may be harmful to the pregnancy – this is an unnecessary fear; sex is not associated with any negative outcomes during pregnancy.

Most of the time discomfort and pain during sex is related to your changing anatomy and body shape. Familiar positions may become uncomfortable because your belly is in the way and more penetrating positions may become less desirable because your uterus has started to take space away from the upper part of your vagina. Usually, a little creativity can be both fun and problem-solving. Rear vaginal-entry positions, with the help of a few pillows or a wedge cushion, can solve several problems at once. The woman on top, if it's not too penetrating, can also be pleasurable for both and it can allow you to determine the angle of entry and the depth of penetration to a degree. Finally, if you lay on your side and draw your top leg upwards, this can allow your partner to straddle your bottom leg and enter at a 90° angle compared to the missionary position. This side saddle approach allows for complete control over the angle of entry and allows you to control the depth of penetration with your top leg.

What can I do for my acne?

Unfortunately, acne tends to get worse during pregnancy. Blame your hormones and your beautiful, oily glow of pregnancy. Still, there are a few things you can do. It is safe to wash your face with benzoyl peroxide during pregnancy. Benzoyl peroxide is the common ingredient in most over-the-counter acne remedies. Check the label and ask your doctor if you're not sure about a particular product.

If you wash your face at night and then go and lay down on your pillow from last night, you may find that you have re-contaminated your face with last night's oils and bacteria. One evidence-based trick is to place a fresh, clean towelette over your pillow each night that you remove in the morning. This towelette can collect the new nightly skin oils and bacteria and not allow them to saturate into your pillow and pillowcase. Just change it each night.

Oral retinoids (e.g., Accutane) should be avoided during pregnancy due to the severity of birth defects that a fetus may develop because of exposure. Many other acne treatments are not safe during pregnancy. Ask your doctor before trying any other remedies.

Why is my heart rate so fast?

Due to some of the physiological changes of pregnancy, it is common for women's resting heart rate to be about 10 to 15 beats per minute faster while pregnant. Pregnant women are also more likely to have bigger increases in their heart rate with exertion since their heart is doing more work while pregnant. This increased work starts in the first trimester, as pregnant women have a blood volume expansion of over 40%. It doesn't stop there, as pregnant women do more work by moving around an extra 30 pounds or more in the third trimester.

As the uterus gets larger, the heart is pushed upwards and rotated to the left. This changing position of the heart allows women to become more aware of their heart beating and sometimes this is alarming because they don't normally perceive that their heart is beating in their chest. Couple this with the fact that the heart may be beating faster than normal, and this can be quite anxiety-provoking. But if your heart rate isn't too fast at rest and you don't notice that it is beating irregularly, don't worry. If you feel like your heart rhythm is irregular or your heart rate is persistently fast and staying that way, talk to your doctor.

I have gestational diabetes. Now what?

If you failed your 1-hour glucose screen AND your 3-hour glucose tolerance test, then you have gestational diabetes.

Hopefully, you'll get a chance to talk to a dietitian. In the meantime, try to cut down (if you can, cut them out completely) the simple sugary items from your diet: colas, cookies, cakes, candies, and other sources of sugary carbs. Paying attention to portion size is the best thing you can do. Try to make your plate ½ greens, ¼ grains, and ¼ protein for every meal. If you're not already, add in four to five 20-minute walks or other cardiovascular exercise sessions per week. Walking after dinner may have the most positive impact on your blood sugars.

You'll need to check your blood sugar several times per day, at least initially. You should check your blood sugar first thing in the morning (a fasting blood glucose) and two hours after each large meal - breakfast, lunch, and dinner. Your fasting blood sugars should be below 95 and your blood sugars two hours after meals should be below 120. If your blood sugars are running higher than this, you may need to take medicine to help lower your blood sugars.

Is also helpful, in the beginning at least, to track what you are eating. This can help your dietitian and your doctor decide if there are some things you should do differently in your diet. It can also help you understand why your blood sugar might spike - for example, after delicious pizza.

Is my discharge normal?

Probably. Pregnant women have more vaginal discharge than nonpregnant women. It is common for pregnant women to wear a panty liner while pregnant because of this discharge. Most of this discharge is physiologic and represents cervical mucus. The more babies you've had, the more likely you are to experience this discharge. If your discharge has a bad odor, itches, or is green, tell your doctor to make sure it's not an infection. Otherwise, expect to have some discharge throughout pregnancy.

Is it normal that my boobs are leaking already?

Yes. Especially if you've already had children, you might notice that your milk comes in early or that you have occasional leakage, even in the first trimester. Even if you haven't had a baby yet, it's not uncommon at all for you to leak some milk. If this is a persistent problem (or an embarrassing one), you might need to change up your bra or wear nipple shields so that your nipples are less stimulated.

Should I hand express/pump after 36 weeks to collect colostrum?

There's no quality scientific evidence that suggests that this is beneficial or harmful. Some women who are anxious about breastfeeding may gain confidence by doing this, but just as many women will suffer pain, frustration, and unnecessary anxiety by attempting to hand express before the baby is born. The highest quality studies have found no health benefits to baby from having colostrum or milk already available at birth.

Can I take baths? Use a hot tub/jacuzzi?

A general rule is to only bathe or soak in water that is comfortable to you. To be specific, we ask that you keep your water temperature below 100-102 °F. The goals of this are:

- Don't burn your skin and
- Don't send yourself into heat stroke/exhaustion.

You should be able to gauge if the temperature of the water you're getting into is going to cause either of these things. No thermometer is needed. If you do like hot baths or showers, just remember that you can get dehydrated quickly and maybe keep cold water and a chair or stool by the tub. Also, get yourself a non-slip bathmat!

Many hot tubs might be set to 104 °F or higher. One study from the 1990s showed that soaking in a hot tub at this higher temperature during the first trimester may be associated with neural tube defects in babies. Because of this study, we recommend avoiding temperatures that high for long periods of time, especially in the first trimester. The research is weak, but it is certainly something to consider.

Hot tubs are different from most baths because the water is maintained at that higher temperature and your body is typically submerged with little opportunity to cool off. But with baths in your home, the water starts to cool immediately after it's drawn so it doesn't raise your core body temperature in the same way or to the same extent as a hot tub might.

Are there cleaning products I should avoid?

Glycol ethers are a type of chemical used in some cleaning products and these should be avoided during pregnancy. Examples of glycol ethers are 2-butoxyethanol (EGBE) and methoxydiglycol (DEGME). Glycol ethers are solvents that have been linked to miscarriage and birth defects. Check the ingredients of the products listed below before you buy them. Here are some products that may contain a glycol ether:

- Resins, lacquers, house paints
- Dyes, inks, some water based paints
- Hydraulic fluids
- Degreasing cleaning agents

A general thing to avoid, not just in pregnancy, is the combination of ammonia and bleach when cleaning because it creates a poisonous gas that can be very harmful to you.

Is it safe to paint?

Paints that contain lead or the above-mentioned glycol ethers should be avoided, but modern paints don't have these substances. Keep the area well ventilated no matter what paints you are using. Other recreational paints for artistic use are generally safe, including watercolors, acrylic, and tempera paints.

I feel like I'm about to pass out! What can I do?

Anything you normally do when you feel that way! Sit or lay down, have someone get you some water and food, and give yourself some time to let the feeling pass. Laying on your left side is best so that your uterus rolls off the blood vessels bringing blood back to your heart. The most important thing is avoiding falling and hurting yourself. As soon as you feel woozy or dizzy, sit or lay down on the ground or in a chair and ask for some help.

Usually, the problem is a lack of blood to your head. When you're pregnant, blood tends to collect in your legs. Your blood vessels relax to allow for increased blood volume and your uterus puts pressure on the vena cava, which is the large vein that drains blood back from your legs to your heart. These factors mean that more blood stays in your legs and has a harder time getting back to your heart. Because of this, there is relatively less blood going to your head sometimes and this may make you feel like you are going to faint.

Blood moves up from your lower extremities with movement of the muscles in your legs. The veins in your legs run through the muscles: when the muscles contract, they squeeze the blood upwards back to your heart, so moving your legs helps move blood upwards whereas standing very still may contribute to blood staying in your legs, lowering the amount of blood returned to your heart, and making you feel light-headed and might even lead to fainting. You might want to wear compression socks to help blood flow and reduce swelling. You should certainly try to maintain good fluid and food intake throughout the day to keep your energy up. Avoid excessive heat like hot showers because your blood vessels will dilate even more when you are hot. A hot shower in the morning could cause you to pass out. A cool rag on the back of your neck may be helpful with these symptoms as well.

Is there a limit to how much I should be lifting?

You shouldn't be worried about lifting general items around the house, the store, or work. If you work on an assembly line in a factory or in some other job that requires routine, repetitive heavy lifting, it may be best to ask your doctor about your specific situation. But for the most part, occasional and recurrent lifting of any amount you normally lift during your home or work life is not usually going to be a problem. This includes any babies or small children you have at home.

Still, lifting the right way is very important: bend at your knees, try to keep your back straight, and lift with your legs. This will help prevent unnecessary strain or sprain on your muscles and joints which are already a bit overworked when you are pregnant.

It's unclear if repetitive heavy lifting is associated with adverse pregnancy outcomes, but it certainly can make the normal aches and pains of pregnancy much worse. At the gym, light weights and repetitions are fine, but it's probably not the time to set your new personal records for lifting.

At work, it depends on how far along you are and how much lifting you do. Scan the QR code for a graphic that shows a very conservative approach to limiting problems associated with repetitive lifting while you're pregnant.

What skin changes are normal and when should I be concerned?

There are lots of skin changes that might happen during pregnancy; some are due to physiologic and hormonal changes, and some are more serious. Let's talk about some common ones.

Spider angiomas. These are little vascular spots that can show up on your skin during pregnancy. They are typically not concerning and will go away when you are no longer pregnant. The only time we would be concerned by them is if you have a history of liver problems or if you begin having symptoms that would be concerning for a liver problem (which is rare).

Linea nigra. This is a normal dark vertical line that can arise from your belly button down towards your pubic bone. It develops because of hormonal changes and will fade away partially once the baby is born. During pregnancy, the placenta develops a hormone called melanocyte-stimulating hormone (MSH). This extra MSH stimulates some cells to make extra melanin which causes these cells to get darker.

Darkened areolae and darkened armpits. There are a lot of changes that may occur with the breasts during pregnancy. The nipples and areolae may become a darker shade due again to extra MSH. Similarly, the color should fade back to near its usual color after the baby is born. While this is completely normal, any redness of the breast should be investigated further by your doctor. The same thing goes for the armpits. You may notice that they are darker and may even look a gray or brown color. This is normal and will fade mostly back to normal once the baby is born.

Melasma. Another case of hyperpigmentation in pregnancy! Are you kidding me?! Are you noticing a theme yet? Unfortunately, this one occurs on the face and women typically do not like it. It will appear as either a gray or brown patchy/spotty change or general change in the coloration of the face. What may be more upsetting to hear is that we don't have a good treatment for it. If it's still present a few months after you've delivered, talk to your doctor about possible treatments. You can prevent it from getting worse by using sun protection like sunscreens, hats, etc. Any sun exposure can make it worse.

Polymorphic eruption of pregnancy (PEP). PEP is a rash of pregnancy that can occur during the third trimester on the abdomen and sometimes upper thighs. This previously was called pruritic urticarial papules and plaques of pregnancy (PUPPP). It will be very itchy and look like plaques, red bumps, or hives. It can start out in the stretch marks and is not harmful to you or baby but can be very annoying for you because of the itchiness. Treatment is a topical steroid cream that your doctor will prescribe for you, and possibly an oral antihistamine (e.g., Benadryl) to control the itch. Cool wet compresses and oatmeal baths may help with the itching.

Pemphigoid gestationis. This rash can occur during the second or third trimester or sometimes right after delivery. This can have similar features to PEP but can extend further on your body beyond the thighs and onto the legs. It may develop blisters as well. The treatment is the same as it is for PEP.

There are some other causes of rash and itching as well, including **atopic eruption of pregnancy** and **pustular psoriasis of pregnancy**. Remember, if your main symptom is intense itching without a rash, be sure to discuss intrahepatic cholestasis of pregnancy with your doctor as this requires medical treatment and earlier delivery.

What does belly measuring tell you?

Belly measuring, or what we call "fundal heights," is a very rough estimate of how the baby is growing throughout the pregnancy. It is the measurement from the top of your uterus (the fundus) to your pubic bone. We expect it to be within about two centimeters from your week gestation starting at 24 weeks. So, for example, at 26 weeks' gestation, the fundal height should be anywhere from 24-28 centimeters.

Many doctors no longer do this test as studies have failed to show that it is accurate or changes pregnancy outcomes. It is a very subjective test, with measurements varying widely from one doctor or midwife to the next, and it is not very sensitive or specific to detect abnormalities in fetal growth. Don't be alarmed if your doctor doesn't measure it! It probably just means she is up to date on the scientific literature.

How do we know if the baby is too big or too small without these measurements? This is largely based on performing ultrasounds for patients who have risk factors for fetal growth abnormalities, such as diabetes, hypertension, obesity or excessive weight gain, and a few other things. We also feel the size of your belly to make sure we are not worried about the baby being too big near the time you deliver. If we are worried, we might order an ultrasound.

Will going to the chiropractor help with aligning things to make for an easier delivery?

Unfortunately, there has not been quality evidence showing that chiropractic alignment will help with delivery. Until there is solid evidence supporting it, we don't recommend it. One thing often recommended is the "Webster technique." This is supposed to ensure that the breech or transverse baby is head down by the end of the pregnancy. Most babies will be head down by 37 weeks or so and this technique is no better than random chance at making sure your baby is head down at term. Don't waste your money.

Does eating six dates a day help soften your cervix for a better labor?

No. If this were the case, we would ask patients to eat dates as their due dates approached and avoid them before that. Alas, there is no evidence to back up this claim. So, eat the dates or don't, but your cervix will do what it is going to do regardless.

Does drinking red raspberry leaf tea, bouncing on a ball, having sex, etc. help start labor?

Babies love being unpredictable. If there were a way to induce labor through drinking tea, eating, dates, exercise, sex, or some other magic, we would tell you. There are dozens of such claims and the reason so many fibs exist is simple: women eventually go into labor and sometimes they will falsely attribute whatever they did immediately prior to labor as the reason things got going. The stronger the correlation of the timing between the onset of labor and the thing they did, the stronger the belief. But the body just does what it is going to do on its own terms. Unless you go into labor spontaneously, the only thing we can do to get it started is induce with medicine.

I drank alcohol before I knew I was pregnant. Is this okay?

This is not an uncommon situation. Many women don't realize they are pregnant and consume alcohol during those early weeks of gestation. Unfortunately, there is no way to diagnose fetal alcohol syndrome until the baby is born. In some severe cases it can be diagnosed right at birth, but most cases are not detected until early childhood, and some very mild cases may not be detected at all.

No amount of alcohol during pregnancy has been deemed safe, and the amount of alcohol consumed is a poor predictor of outcomes. The only way we can determine the effects of any alcohol consumption you might have had is by assessing the child during their development and seeing how they are doing with their cognitive, behavioral, and other developmental milestones. It is best to try and avoid alcohol when you are thinking about conceiving. Once you find out you are pregnant, cut out alcohol entirely and avoid it for the rest of the pregnancy if you have not already done so.

How can I quit smoking?

Cutting out smoking completely is very difficult for most patients, but doing so can drastically reduce the risks to your pregnancy and your own health. There are several **nicotine replacement therapies (NRT)** such as: nicotine gum, patches, tablets, lozenges, inhalers (not the same thing as a vape), sprays, and strips. We also have medications that can help with the urges.

E-cigarettes are not a good option because they are not licensed or controlled for safety in pregnancy, and we have no evidence that they are any safer in the long-term than cigarettes.

Giving up smoking cold turkey is hard. If you can give yourself time to quit gradually during the time when you are trying to get pregnant, this might be more effective. This involves reducing the number of cigarettes you smoke by one or two every week until you are completely off cigarettes.

If you are pregnant and trying to stop smoking, you can also try substituting cigarettes with one of the NRTs mentioned above. This could mean using a patch and quitting all cigarettes or using an inhaler or gum and replacing a single cigarette here and there as you cut down. The goal is to get you to stop and stop for good, rather than quit for a week and then fall off the bandwagon and start up all over again. When you are tempted to smoke, try the following:

- Delay the act of smoking as long as you can
- Deep breaths
- Drink water
- Do something else (something with your hands is best)

Why am I peeing so much?

In the first trimester, certain hormones your pregnant body makes can stimulate urine production and the urge to pee. As the baby grows and the uterus expands, the bladder, located directly in front of the uterus, gets compressed. This means the bladder probably holds less urine before you develop the urge to pee. These forces conspire together to make pregnant women pee a million times a day. It is important to remember that if you feel you are peeing an unusual amount with burning, you might have a UTI.

What can help you stop peeing so much, you ask? First, don't stop drinking fluids. You need them to stay hydrated! But you can cut down on them two to three hours before you go to bed to avoid so many nighttime interruptions. Avoiding caffeinated drinks also helps. In the third trimester, try positional changes to avoid compression of the bladder by the uterus.

These mood swings are crazy. Help!

Mood swings are common in pregnancy and may be self-limited. Pregnant women are tired, often anxious about the pregnancy and the changes of life occurring and are busy preparing for a new baby. There isn't too much we can do for you here. But it is important to distinguish an occasional mood swing from depression or anxiety. If you feel like your mood swings are uncontrollable and very bad, you should discuss them with your doctor so they can make sure that something more serious isn't going on. The best way to take care of perinatal mental health problems is by catching and addressing them early. Many pregnant women, however, have some overwhelming moments but don't necessarily have an underlying mood disorder like depression or anxiety.

One of the best things to do for these types of mood swings is personal soothing techniques. This might mean setting aside some personal time during your day or week, talking to your friends and family about things they can do to help you, or finding a confidant or therapist. Pregnancy is stressful and the physical and psychological toll can be immense. Support and advice from others can help tremendously.

Mood swings are a part of pregnancy. There are a lot of changes going on with your body and your life. It is important to know that you can do this, and your doctor and support system should be there to help you every step of the way.

Why am I having weird dreams?

REM (rapid eye movement) sleep is the term we use for deep restful sleep when people experience vivid dreams. Pregnant women experience more REM sleep and therefore may feel like they have more vivid dreams as well as more frequent dreams. Their sleep is also disrupted more often due to things like discomfort, restless legs, frequent urination, etc. Restless sleep can also lead to an increase in hypnagogic hallucinations, which are the abnormal sensations that occur right as you are falling asleep (like a sensation of falling, strange smells, etc.).

The result of all of this is that pregnant women tend to remember more of their dreams. Sometimes, our anxieties play themselves out in dream scenarios so it's not uncommon for your dreams to contain content that might be disturbing (things like losing the pregnancy or your child being hurt or injured in some way). If you find that the content of your dreams is particularly disturbing, talk to your doctor.

Let's Have A Baby!

How can I tell if I'm in labor?

Every pregnant woman at some point in her pregnancy will begin to wonder if she is in labor. Most women have a few false starts. Braxton-Hicks contractions can be confusing and can become frequent and regular – at least for a short time – before going back to their irregular pattern. Women frequently have physiologic discharge or will urinate and wonder if their water is broken. So how can you tell real labor from false labor?

The answer is time. Real labor is progressive in every way, but you won't be able to see this until some time has passed. If you're having regular contractions, the best thing to do is see what happens over the next two to three hours. If you are really in labor, your contractions will become more frequent (maybe going from every six to seven minutes apart to every three to four minutes apart), last longer (going from, say, 30 seconds in length to 45 or 50 seconds in length), become more painful, regular, predictable, and persistent. False labor, on the other hand, may start strong but will lose steam and wane over two to three hours.

If it's your first baby, you have plenty of time. Labor will likely last many hours and you will have plenty of time to arrive at the hospital. If it's your fourth baby, then you already know what to expect. If you are reading this anyway, your labor probably won't last that long, and you should head to the hospital a little sooner.

In some cases, your doctor may ask you to come to the hospital a bit earlier; for example, if you're positive for group B Streptococcus, then you will need four hours of IV antibiotic therapy in addition to however long it takes to get to the hospital, get admitted, and get an IV started before the baby is born.

If your water breaks, you should probably head to the hospital. This may be a sign that your labor is already very advanced, since water tends to break on its own at an average of about 8 cm. If your water is broken and you're not already in labor, then you should still go to the hospital because your labor likely needs to be augmented or induced.

If you have had a previous Cesarean delivery, then you should come to the hospital much sooner because you do not want to risk laboring at home. A trial of labor after Cesarean is a good idea for most women, but because of the risk of uterine rupture, that trial of labor should happen at the hospital to maximize the safety of mom and baby.

What does losing my mucus plug mean?

Many women will pass a large plug of mucus (and maybe some blood) at some point during cervical dilation. As the cervix dilates and thins, the mucus buildup that was there in the cervical canal can come out. It has also been called "the bloody show" if it's blood tinged.

Losing this plug doesn't have any diagnostic or predictive value for us as doctors. Many people think "it's go time" when they lose it or that they are going to progress faster after its expulsion. However, women can start to dilate a small amount early and lose it even weeks before they go into labor. Sorry to disappoint you, but the baby is going to come when it's ready.

Is my water broken?

You can't always tell; but, in general, once your water breaks, it keeps coming. Ruptured membranes are not just a small gush or a little bit of spotting; if you think your water has broken, clean up and see if the leakage persists. If it does or you are unsure, you probably need to be examined.

Discharge is common in pregnancy but usually never results in more leakage than would fill a small pad or panty liner. If you are getting cervical checks at your later appointments, the gel we use can sometimes appear later as a leakage of fluid, but it is usually only a small amount, and you would not see continued leakage.

Probably the most common reason why women believe that their water has broken is because they have peed on themselves. Most women cannot believe that they have peed on themselves, especially if they never felt the urge to pee, but in the third trimester with the baby's head smashed right against the bladder, this is a common occurrence. If it happens on your bed sheets or in your underwear, you won't always be able to tell that it is urine by smell or color alone. Amniotic fluid has a unique odor that is like a combination of ejaculate and bleach; that may not be helpful if you've never smelled amniotic fluid before, but when you do, maybe you'll recognize it.

Still, large gushes with continual leakage after the fact should be assessed at the hospital or your doctor's office. You may be ready to rock and roll!

What should I bring in my hospital bag?

This is a preference thing. There is no right or wrong answer here. You are not required to bring anything aside from your ID and insurance card if you have them. The rest of your bag should be things that bring you comfort.

If you do a labor and delivery tour at some point before you deliver (most hospitals offer this), you can ask what amenities they have that you may want (labor tub, birthing balls, fan, etc.). If they do not have these things, then you may want to bring them.

Things the hospital will provide: sanitary pads for you after delivery, diapers, formula, bottle nipples, food/drink, gowns, and hygiene products for showering.

Things you may want: phone charger, socks, snacks, your own clothes/robe/toiletries that you prefer, multiple changes of clothes (you may be very sweaty/uncomfortable during the labor period), slippers, shower shoes (hospital showers should be clean - but still), etc. Think about going away on a trip to a hotel for 3 days or so and pack whatever you would take for that.

When will the doctor check my cervix?

There's no reason to check your cervix unless you're having signs of labor, like regular contractions, bleeding, or leakage of fluid. If you're considering an induction, checking your cervix might be helpful to see if your cervix is favorable. If your cervix isn't ready for labor (not dilated at all), then an induction might unnecessarily increase your chances of a Cesarean delivery.

Do I need cervical checks during labor?

Cervical check frequency can vary by hospital. It is true that more cervical checks lead to an increased risk of infection. However, some checks are necessary to determine labor progress. We can optimize the risk/benefit ratio. Checking every two hours is common in some hospitals but is usually not necessary. In the latent phase of labor, from 0-6 cm, checking every *X* number of hours is not necessary. If you are being induced and you have a cervical ripening agent in place, like a cervical medication or a catheter balloon, then at the time of placement you are checked and the next check should occur when a decision is being made: for example, do you need another dose of medication, or can the catheter be removed? This may be many hours (usually at least four).

How often the cervix is checked should be based on patient feedback (feeling more pressure, contractions getting stronger/closer together, etc.), and usually no more often than every four hours in latent labor. Even in active labor, from 6-10 cm, we don't worry about "failure to progress" until four hours of no cervical change. Therefore, we can check at four hours and usually still have all the information necessary to determine if something should be done about slow labor.

Remember, sometimes there can be a good reason to check more often, especially if you get towards the end and continue to feel a lot of pressure or even begin feeling the urge to push. We want to check you as few times as necessary while still making sure we can monitor your progress.

When can I get induced?

Inductions happen for lots of good reasons – but also some not so good ones. Unless there's a medical reason to do so, you shouldn't be induced before 39 weeks' gestation. Even at 39 weeks, induction might not be the best idea unless your body is ready for labor. Checking your cervix can help determine this. Otherwise, it might be better to wait until 41 weeks. After 41 weeks' gestation, it's unusual that going any further makes much sense due to increasing risks for the baby and no benefit to the mother in terms of decreased Cesarean rate (in fact, the risk of Cesarean goes up after 41 weeks' gestation).

Sometimes you might need to be induced much earlier, but it should be because you have a medical problem like high blood pressure or some other complication.

Will I need an episiotomy?

No! Except in some very rare emergency cases, episiotomies should never be performed. If your doctor performs routine or frequent episiotomies, then he may not be practicing up-to-date medicine. We have known since the mid-1980s that episiotomies are harmful and unnecessary except in a handful of rare emergencies, such as severe shoulder dystocia.

This doesn't mean that you might not tear, but however badly you might tear, an episiotomy likely would have made the tear much worse.

Does perineal massage help prevent tears?

Perineal massage a few weeks leading up to delivery may decrease the chance that you tear, but it does so by causing unwanted (and permanent) relaxation of the vaginal tissues. It isn't worth it. During labor, your doctor or midwife may provide some slight pressure on the perineum while you are complete and pushing. This can be seen as a massage, but we are just helping to slowly stretch some of those muscles in the pelvic floor as the head begins to descend. This encourages the tissues to relax rather than contract right back after a contraction and pull the baby back in after the progress you just made with your pushing. At the actual moment of crowning of the baby's head, studies have shown that a grip of the perineal tissues (applying counterpressure to the stretch of those tissues) can help prevent significant tears at the time the head delivers out of the vagina – the moment when most tears occur.

Am I going to poop during delivery?

You might, but don't worry about it. We are all used to it and completely unfazed by it. If you ask us if you did, we will probably lie to you and say no (the only lie you will hear from us, we promise). The reality is that you have a big head pushing down right against your rectum while you're pushing. In fact, we tell you that the pushing you do to deliver the baby should feel like "the biggest poop of your life," because you are directing all that pressure down towards your bottom. If it happens, then you're pushing in the right spot! It will be wiped away and no one will have a second thought about it.

Is there a best way to push?

The most effective pushing is usually done when you take in a deep breath, fill up your lungs, and then hold that air in while you bear down, tuck your chin to your chest, and push as hard as you can into your bottom. We encourage you to hold those breaths for 10 seconds and attempt two to three rounds of 10 seconds of pushing if the contraction allows it and you are able. Typically, the moms that scream or let the air out tend to have less effective pushing. When the lungs are filled with air, they push the diaphragm down, increasing your internal abdominal pressure, which helps with the pushing force. Still, feel free to scream, cry, or do whatever you need to do to get through it. No one is judging you. The reality is, labor can be a long process, and your doctor can give you feedback on what pushing methods you should try to yield the best result.

The position you're in while pushing can vary widely. When you lay on your back and pull your legs back, MRI studies have shown that this creates the most space for the baby. That is not what is commonly claimed by a lot of birth advocates who argue for pushing while squatting or in some other upright position. However, those positions tend to put pressure on the lateral sides of the pelvis (at your hips) and make the pelvis wider but narrower from front to back, which is where it really matters.

The truth is women should be allowed to push in whatever position they are most comfortable and different positions will provide different degrees of pain relief. We will help you know if your pushing is effective and if you might be better served pushing in a different position.

Will I need a Cesarean?

We hope not! But some women do, of course. Cesarean delivery is overused in the United States. There are some good reasons why a woman might need one:

- If she has had a prior "classical" Cesarean delivery (where the incision on the uterus is made higher than normal)
- If she has had **more than two** prior regular ("low transverse" incision) Cesareans

- If she has placenta previa (where the placenta covers or is very close to the cervix) or vasa previa (where placental blood vessels cover the cervix)
- If her baby is breech or sideways (and the doctor is unable to turn the baby to be head-down)
- If her baby does not tolerate labor (this should be relatively rare and there are some specific criteria that can indicate this)
- If her baby is too big, which is more than 5,000 grams (or about 11 lbs.) for a nondiabetic mother or more than 4,500 grams (or just under 9 lbs. 15 oz) for a diabetic mother
- If her labor doesn't progress or she is unable to push the baby out after sufficient time (many doctors don't give women enough time for these things; however, we have criteria we can follow to determine if this is happening)
- If she has triplets, quadruplets (or more), or monochorionic-monoamniotic twins
- If she has active genital herpes or uncontrolled HIV

Those are just about all the reasons, aside from the more emergent ones we won't go into here. We don't know for sure, but as many as half of all Cesareans performed are unnecessary. Most of the unnecessary Cesareans are related to impatience. Guidelines from the American College of Obstetricians and Gynecologists (ACOG) will, if followed, result in significantly fewer Cesareans.

Should I have a water birth?

Probably not. This is a trick question, though. You must separate out laboring in the water and giving birth in water. Most of the known advantages of water birth are related to the process of laboring in water while the known disadvantages of water birth are associated with giving birth in the water.

For example, the benefits of reduced pain during the first stage of labor (that is, the part leading up to pushing), a shorter first stage of labor, and less need for anesthesia all occur before the birth itself takes place. At the same time, the reported disadvantages of a water birth all take place during the actual process of delivery, including newborn aspiration, drowning, infections, hyponatremia, depressed Apgar scores, and umbilical cord rupture. So, it probably makes the most sense to labor in the water and then get out on dry land when it's time to push and have the baby.

If you think about it, nature designed the birth process to happen on dry land. One of the benefits of a vaginal delivery compared to a Cesarean delivery is that the baby gets most of the amniotic fluid squeezed out of her lungs while traveling through the birth canal so that her first breath, once delivered, is full of nice, clean air. This doesn't always happen with a Cesarean delivery and, consequently, babies have higher rates of respiratory problems with Cesarean birth as compared to vaginal birth. In any event, when a baby is born vaginally underwater, the first inspiration by the baby may be underwater and therefore lead to aspiration of water with subsequent increased risk of infections, drowning, and other respiratory problems.

Keep these things in mind when you read about water births being more natural than land births. There's nothing natural about it at all. In fact, water births are a rather modern invention. Currently, the American Academy of Pediatrics and the American College of Obstetricians and Gynecologists recommend against deliveries occurring underwater.

Should I VBAC?

If you've had a previous Cesarean delivery (or two), you may be a candidate for a trial of labor after Cesarean (TOLAC). This is a complicated issue. The short answer is that most women with only one prior cesarean delivery should try VBAC (vaginal birth after Cesarean), but you should read more about it in the next few pages.

Should I store my baby's cord blood?

The reality of cord blood banking is that it is a huge expense for little to no benefit for the average person. Private cord blood banking has an initial collection fee anywhere from $1,000-$2,000 and then an annual storage fee that can be around $200 per year, depending on the bank. Cord blood contains stem cells that can be beneficial in the treatment of different blood and bone marrow disorders. If there is a family history of a disease with a known genetic component, then there may be an argument for storing it, but not everyone has the money and not every disease can be predicted so you must weigh the risks and benefits for your situation.

There is very little research involving stem cell therapies that involve using blood from umbilical cords and there is a real concern over how many stem cells can be retrieved from these frozen samples after a few years in the freezer. It is questionable if any child so far has ever benefited from having cord blood frozen, so it's probably best to keep it limited to a few rare situations involving some rather rare diseases or as part of a research protocol.

What is delayed cord clamping and what length of time is best?

After the baby is born, there should be a pause before clamping the cord (as opposed to immediately clamping it). This is called **delayed cord clamping** or **optimal cord clamping**. The baby is placed on your chest/belly depending on the length of the cord and if the baby appears healthy, your doctor will wait at least 60 seconds OR until the baby gets their first good cry before clamping and cutting the cord and detaching the baby from the placenta. Studies have shown that at least 60 seconds is optimal, but longer than that is okay as well. The baby can get an additional 80 mL of blood during this time. That extra blood has been shown to improve hemoglobin and iron stores within the first year of life, and improve cognitive, motor, and behavioral development. After this, the doctor will clamp the cord and hand someone of your choosing the scissors to cut the cord. Then, while you pay attention to your new baby, the placenta will be delivered with gentle traction, and you will no longer be pregnant!

Delayed cord clamping is the standard of care and has been for several years.

Should I have a home birth?

Well, you'll think we're biased for saying it, but the answer is no. While birth can be (and usually is) a very benign event, the truth is that the safest place for you to deliver is in a hospital. It is the safest option for your and your baby's health in case anything goes wrong. We cannot completely predict who will have issues at the time of delivery or leading up to it. We know of certain risk factors that increase the chance of serious events happening, but ultimately, several things could happen to even the healthiest people.

The biggest risk factor for issues at delivery, believe it or not, is being nulliparous (a woman who has not delivered a child before). The reasoning behind this is because we do not know if you have an adequate pelvis for childbirth and you are at the greatest risk for shoulder dystocia and stalled labor. In the next section, we discuss some complications that can arise during pregnancy. One thing that all these complications have in common is that the quicker we identify them and come up with a plan to treat them, the better it is for you and your baby. That identification and treatment is best facilitated if you are in a hospital under the care of nurses and physicians that can monitor for these things.

The bottom line is that studies consistently show that even with low-risk and well-selected patients, home birth is consistently more dangerous for mom and baby.

Details about the hospital

Giving birth is a natural process but it is still associated with certain risks to you and your baby. Your doctors and nurses will work together with you to provide the least invasive and safest environment possible for you and your baby. Please read the following information regarding the labor and delivery process and certain risks and benefits associated with procedures sometimes used during labor; then, discuss any questions you may have with your doctor.

Spontaneous vaginal delivery. This term refers to normal, vaginal childbirth. This is our goal for you during your labor. If you desire, we can provide you with different options for pain control including pain medications in your IV, local anesthetic in your perineum or near the pudendal nerves in your vagina, epidural anesthesia, or, in many hospitals, inhaled nitrous oxide. Your anesthesia provider will discuss the risks and benefits of an epidural with you before proceeding if you choose that option. If you do not want any of these things, that is totally fine! Just know that you have options.

Augmentation. In some cases, your labor may become slowed or stop altogether, and it may be necessary to use a medicine called **oxytocin (Pitocin)**. This will make your contractions stronger and closer together. Rarely, this medicine can cause your contractions to become too strong or too close together, which may stress your baby. In almost all cases, this risk is easily manageable, and we can decrease the contractions by turning down or turning off the medicine or by using another medicine called terbutaline (Brethine) to stop the contractions in emergencies.

In rare cases, it is necessary to perform an **emergency Cesarean delivery** for the safety of the baby. The risks of not using oxytocin to augment a stalled or slowed labor, however, include an increased risk of Cesarean delivery for arrest of labor, an increased risk of an infection in your uterus or your baby, a longer labor, and a risk of maternal exhaustion that leads to more Cesareans or operative deliveries.

Amniotomy. Another method of augmenting your labor is called amniotomy or breaking water. This is done during a vaginal exam with a small plastic hook and benefits include a decreased risk of Cesarean delivery, shorter labors, less need for oxytocin, and the ability to monitor the baby's heartbeat and your contractions with internal monitors, if needed. Risks are very small, but not absent, and include an increased risk of infection, a very small risk of the umbilical cord falling through the cervix requiring emergency Cesarean delivery, and the plastic hook can leave a small scratch on the baby's head in some cases.

Induction of labor. Sometimes, if labor has not started on its own, it may be necessary to induce labor for the well-being of the baby and/or mother. Induction can be carried out many ways and depends on several factors, including the reason for induction, your obstetrical history, and your cervical exam. In many cases, induction can be carried out only with oxytocin and/or amniotomy, as discussed above. However, in some cases, the cervix needs to be ripened. Cervical ripening is usually accomplished with medications called prostaglandins, including **misoprostol (Cytotec)** or **dinoprostone (Cervidil)**, or with balloons placed through the cervix. Like oxytocin, these medications can occasionally make contractions too strong or too frequent, and emergent Cesarean delivery may, rarely, be necessary because of fetal distress. Overall, however, your risk of Cesarean delivery is higher if these drugs are not used when they are necessary. Some women who might have had a vaginal delivery if her labor started on its own will need a Cesarean delivery after a failed induction attempt, so it is important to discuss with your doctor the specific reasons for induction.

Monitoring. Normally during labor, a nurse will place monitors on your abdomen to measure the frequency of your contractions and to monitor the fetal heartbeat. Occasionally, it is necessary to use monitors placed in the vagina. An **intrauterine pressure catheter (IUPC)** can be placed through the vagina into a space between the wall of your uterus and the fetal head to measure how strong your contractions are. Insertion of an IUPC is very safe but, rarely, may cause an infection in your uterus and, very rarely, may cause bleeding from the placenta or an early separation of the placenta, called an abruption. This can cause stress for the baby and might require a Cesarean delivery. Sometimes a monitor called a **fetal scalp electrode (FSE)** is placed through the vagina onto the baby's head to record the baby's heartbeat more accurately. Occasionally, this can cause a small scab on the baby's head after birth, and it may rarely cause a superficial infection on the baby's head. Fetal monitoring, whether externally or internally, does not prevent cerebral palsy or birth defects. If you are low-risk and in spontaneous labor, you may be a candidate for **intermittent monitoring**, where the fetal heart rate is listened to every 15 minutes while in labor and every five minutes while pushing, instead of continuous monitoring.

Amnioinfusion. Sometimes, a non-reassuring pattern in the fetal heart tracing can be corrected with a technique called amnioinfusion, where sterile saline is infused through an IUPC into your uterus, relieving pressure off the umbilical cord. This is associated with an increased risk of infection in your uterus but may prevent some Cesarean deliveries.

Tears/episiotomy. During birth, many women (reported to be upwards of 80%) get small tears around the vaginal opening and some will get larger tears in the perineum that, in rare cases, may extend into the rectum. Rarely, it is necessary to cut an episiotomy during some emergencies to help deliver your baby, and cutting an episiotomy carries a greater risk of tears extending into the rectum. Sometimes tears happen in the walls of the vagina or in the cervix. Most of these tears are unavoidable. Some of them will require dissolvable stitches. The areas torn may be swollen and painful for a few days and very rarely these areas may become infected. You may have burning with urination. More severe tears and tears that extend into the rectum are associated with an increased risk of fecal incontinence and pain during intercourse later in life, but most women do not have these problems.

Local anesthetics/pudendal block. Sometimes, if you do not have an epidural or if your epidural does not provide adequate pain relief, it will be necessary to inject a local anesthetic into the area around your vaginal opening to repair tears or lacerations. Occasionally, a special injection of local anesthetic near the pudendal nerves just inside your vagina can provide pain relief at the end of your labor. Injection of local anesthetics are associated with rare allergic reactions or injection into large blood vessels could rarely cause an abnormal maternal heartbeat. Very rarely, a serious infection can occur with the placement of a pudendal nerve block. The benefits of local anesthetics or pudendal nerve block include pain relief, and sometimes a pudendal nerve block can allow delivery with a vacuum or forceps that would prevent a Cesarean delivery.

Operative vaginal delivery. About 10% of women require some assistance by the doctor to deliver the baby through the birth canal. This is done either by means of a **vacuum-assisted vaginal delivery (VAVD)** or **forceps-assisted vaginal delivery (FAVD).** These types of deliveries may be necessary because of problems with the baby's heartbeat or because you are unable to push because of a medical problem, fatigue, or if pushing alone has not been enough to deliver the baby. Forceps and vacuums may cause tears in the vagina, cervix, or perineum, including severe tears into the rectum. Both can cause bleeding under the baby's scalp and very rarely this bleeding can be serious. Forceps can also cause a temporary paralysis of the baby's facial muscles. Very rarely, this can become permanent, though often this type of facial nerve palsy is due to a developmental abnormality. Vacuums usually cause a bruise and bump on the baby's head where the plastic suction cup was applied, called a chignon. This usually disappears in about a week. Very rarely, a vacuum can cause a tear in the baby's scalp. Benefits of both types of operative vaginal delivery include a decreased need for Cesarean delivery and the ability to speed up delivery when the baby may be distressed. If, however, a forceps or vacuum delivery is unsuccessful, an emergent Cesarean delivery will be necessary.

Shoulder dystocia. In about 1% of births, the baby's shoulders do not deliver easily after the head has passed through the birth canal. This is called shoulder dystocia. Your doctor may have to perform several different maneuvers designed to deliver your baby as safely as possible. Shoulder dystocia is associated with a risk of a broken collarbone or arm and sometimes damage to the nerves of the baby's shoulder can occur either during pushing or during maneuvers to free your baby's shoulders. This nerve injury, called a brachial plexus injury, is usually temporary and will get better either on its own or with physical therapy. Rarely, the injury is permanent, leading to permanent dysfunction of the affected arm. The baby may also be at risk for brain damage due to a lack of oxygen while the baby is stuck. When injuries to the arm or collarbone occur, it is often because your doctor is trying to prevent permanent injury to your baby's brain or death. Unfortunately, we cannot predict which babies will have a shoulder dystocia. Risk factors include large babies, mothers who are diabetic or obese, and slow labors combined with the use of forceps or a vacuum. However, in most cases where these factors exist, no shoulder dystocia occurs. What's more, most shoulder dystocias happen with either only one risk factor or no risk factors present, so we have no reliable way of predicting who will experience this complication. If your baby is very large, your doctor may recommend Cesarean delivery to prevent shoulder dystocia (more than 5,000 grams for most women or more than 4,500 grams for diabetic women).

Placenta. After delivery of your baby, the placenta (or afterbirth) must also be delivered. This usually happens just a few minutes after the delivery of your baby and is rarely associated with problems. The nurse will start oxytocin during this time to help your uterus contract down and prevent unnecessary bleeding after delivery. However, sometimes excessive bleeding does occur, called **postpartum hemorrhage**. If this happens, your doctors may order additional oxytocin or other medications, called uterotonics, to help stop the bleeding. Rarely, a blood transfusion is necessary, and this can be associated with an allergic reaction or about a 1 in 2,000,000 chance of serious infections such as Hepatitis C or HIV. You need to tell your doctor if you are unwilling to accept a blood transfusion to save your life. In very rare cases of postpartum hemorrhage, as a live-saving measure, it is necessary for your doctor to perform emergency surgery to control the bleeding, and very rarely, this may include performing an emergency hysterectomy (removal of the uterus).

Sometimes, the placenta does not deliver on its own and your doctor may have to perform manual extraction of the placenta. In this procedure, your doctor will deliver the placenta with her hand placed in your uterus. This increases your risk of an infection in the uterus but decreases the risk of serious bleeding. Very rarely, because the placenta cannot be delivered, it is necessary to perform a **D&C (dilation and curettage)**, where instruments are used, under anesthesia, to detach and remove the placenta from your uterus. This increases your risk of a blood transfusion as well as your risk of infection. Occasionally, the instruments used can perforate your uterus causing damage to the organs around your uterus, such as the bowel or bladder, and your doctor may need to perform emergency surgery to repair these organs.

Infections. Occasionally, an infection may occur while you are in labor, or before labor, particularly if your water has broken. This infection is called **chorioamnionitis**. Your doctor will start antibiotics if this happens and treat your fever. However, your baby may be born with a serious infection if this occurs. Sometimes, Cesarean delivery is necessary because of stress to your baby. Also, an infection may occur after your delivery called **endometritis**. This also may require antibiotics. Your doctor will try to limit factors that may put you at risk for infection, but not all infections are preventable.

All these risks we've been discussing are, fortunately, relatively rare and we are typically good at preventing and treating them when they do occur. We try everything in our power to make the birth experience a smooth one for you. That being said, we want you to be informed every step of the way.

Understand the risks of a Cesarean delivery

Nearly one-third of babies today are born by Cesarean delivery, where the doctor delivers the baby through an incision in the abdomen and uterus. Reasons for a Cesarean include repeat Cesareans for women with one or more prior Cesareans; breech or transverse presentation of your baby; arrested labor or cephalopelvic disproportion (where either the baby is too big, or the maternal pelvis is too small for safe delivery to occur); fetal distress (where the baby will not tolerate normal labor safely); and other less common reasons. Sometimes, Cesareans are planned and occur on a scheduled basis *before* labor has started; but sometimes Cesareans are emergent and occur *after* labor has started. In general, planned Cesareans are safer for the mother and baby than emergent Cesareans. There are, of course, unique risks to Cesarean delivery, which are discussed below.

Bleeding. There will almost always be more bleeding at the time of a Cesarean delivery than with a vaginal delivery. A blood transfusion is needed about 1 in 80 times. In about 1 in 700 births, it is necessary to perform a hysterectomy. This is often done as a life-saving measure because of otherwise uncontrollable bleeding and would mean that you could not become pregnant again. The risk of hysterectomy for bleeding increases with the risk of something we call placenta accreta spectrum disorders, the risk of which increases with the number of repeat Cesarean deliveries.

Infection. Infection in your uterus, abdomen, or incision can follow a Cesarean delivery. Usually, infections in the uterus can be treated easily with antibiotics. Antibiotics which are given at the time of your Cesarean don't guarantee that you won't get an infection. Occasionally, an infection in your wound will require it to be opened and debrided and it may take some time for the wound to heal. Very rarely, an infection in your abdomen, called an abscess, will require additional surgery.

Damage to other organs. During less than 1% of Cesareans, the organs around the uterus may be damaged. This includes the bladder, bowel, ovaries, fallopian tubes, and ureters (the tubes running from the kidneys to the bladder). Most of the time, these injuries are found at the time of surgery. If this happens, your doctor will do whatever is necessary at the time to repair the injury. These types of injuries are more common in women who have had previous Cesareans or previous surgery in their abdomen or pelvis.

Blood clots. About 1 in 300 women will have a blood clot in her legs following a Cesarean that requires treatment with blood thinners, and sometimes this blood clot can move to the lungs, which can be fatal. Blood clots are more common following a Cesarean than a vaginal delivery. Your doctor will ask you to walk soon and often following your delivery to try to prevent blood clots from forming.

Injury to the baby. Less than 1% of the time, the baby can be injured during your Cesarean. Usually, these injuries are very minor - often a small, shallow cut. Occasionally, the baby might have a broken arm or collarbone, although this is more likely to happen with a vaginal delivery than a Cesarean delivery.

Ileus. Occasionally, following a Cesarean, bowel function is slow to return. This usually only lasts two to three days. It is okay to use stool softeners like Dulcolax or extra fiber or MiraLAX to help things get moving.

Anesthesia. Most women (about 95%) have either a spinal or epidural for anesthesia, allowing the mother to remain awake during her surgery. Sometimes, circumstances require general anesthesia, where the mother is put to sleep. Your nurse anesthetist and/or anesthesiologist will discuss the risks and benefits of these types of anesthesia with you in detail.

Risks in future pregnancies. Some risks of Cesarean delivery are not realized until later pregnancies. One is the risk of the scar on the uterus rupturing in subsequent labors. This risk is generally less than 1%, depending on how many Cesareans you have had. This risk may be even higher if you have what is called a "classical Cesarean delivery," where a vertical incision is made on the uterus (rather than the horizontal or transverse incision that is usually used). This may be necessary if your baby is very small or if it turns in a way that makes it difficult to deliver. Another is the risk of the placenta becoming abnormally attached to the uterus (placenta accreta). This risk increases with each Cesarean you have.

Death. Although pregnancy and childbirth are very safe compared to most medical conditions, it unfortunately can still lead to maternal death about one time in every 10,000 births. Causes for this include severe bleeding, blood clots in the lungs, hypertension, and other medical problems the mother may have. Also, some babies do not survive birth or have significant problems after birth, particularly if they are born very early or are very small. About six to seven babies out of 1,000 die late in pregnancy either before birth or shortly afterward due to a variety of problems with the baby or mother. Many of these deaths cannot be predicted or prevented, but if you or your baby are at a higher risk for problems, your doctor will work closely with you to provide extra surveillance and testing for you and your baby.

Choosing between a repeat Cesarean and a trial of labor after Cesarean (TOLAC)

After Cesarean delivery, a woman may choose to have a planned Cesarean birth or choose a trial of labor for vaginal birth. It is likely that 60-80% of women who try a **vaginal birth after Cesarean (VBAC)** delivery will be successful. We want you to understand the benefits and risks of your choices. There is some amount of risk that goes along with every pregnancy. These risks are greater for women who have had a prior Cesarean delivery. We share the same goal as you: a healthy baby delivered to a healthy mom. We will make every effort to ensure this.

What are the benefits of successful VBAC compared to a planned Cesarean birth?

- Faster time to heal after birth
- Shorter hospital stay
- Less risk of infection after delivery
- Less chance of blood transfusions
- No chance of complications caused by surgery (infection, injury to bowel or urinary tract, or blood loss)
- Less risk that the baby will have breathing problems
- Quicker return to normal activities because there is no pain from surgery
- Greater chance of having a vaginal birth in future pregnancies

- Less risk of problems with how the placenta attaches in future pregnancies
- Higher rates of successful breastfeeding

What are the risks of VBAC?

- A tear or opening in the uterus (womb) occurs in **5 to 10 women out of every 1,000** low risk women who try VBAC (0.5% to 1.0%).

Risks to the mother if there is a tear in the uterus include:

- Blood loss that may need transfusion
- Damage to the uterus that may need hysterectomy (removal of the uterus)
- Damage to the bladder
- Infection
- Death (which is very rare)

Not all tears in the uterus harm the baby. About 7% of the time the baby is harmed when the uterus tears. The most important risks to the baby if there is a tear of the uterus are brain damage and death. In other words, 5 to 10 babies out of every 10,000 VBAC tries will suffer brain damage or death (0.05% to 0.1%) due to uterine rupture.

The risk of your uterus tearing during labor is slightly increased with any of the following:

- Labor that is induced (does not start on its own)
- More than 1 prior Cesarean delivery
- Less than 18 months since your last Cesarean delivery
- An infection at the time of your previous Cesarean

Normal risks of having a vaginal birth are also present for a successful VBAC.

Other risks for the uterus tearing are being researched. Most, but not all, studies have found a slight increased risk for uterine tearing if oxytocin is required to increase the strength or frequency of the uterine contractions during labor that started naturally (spontaneous labor). According to the American College of Obstetricians and Gynecologists, it is still acceptable to VBAC even if you've had two prior Cesareans, a larger baby, or twins.

What are the risks of an unsuccessful VBAC?

- If a vaginal birth cannot occur, then a Cesarean birth must be done. Overall, 60-80% of attempted VBACs are successful.
- A Cesarean delivery after attempting vaginal delivery has the same types of risks as a planned Cesarean delivery.

In addition, some of the risks of surgery are increased (compared to a planned Cesarean delivery) if a Cesarean is needed after an unsuccessful VBAC trial. These risks include:

- Infection
- Transfusion
- Blood clots in the legs or lungs
- Hysterectomy

What are the risks of a planned Cesarean birth if that is my choice?

- The risk that the uterus will tear before a planned Cesarean birth is 2 in 1,000 (0.2%). Because you have a scar on your uterus from your prior Cesarean birth, you will always be at risk for having a tear in your uterus. The tears usually occur during labor but can occur without labor.
- Blood loss and possible blood transfusions. This risk may not differ between planned vaginal birth and planned Cesarean birth.
- More scars developing on the uterus. Women with more than two prior Cesarean deliveries are not offered VBAC trials because of the increasing risk of uterine rupture during labor.
- Infection possibly requiring additional hospital days and IV antibiotics.
- Scarring inside the abdomen.
- Injury to organs inside the body.
- Problems with anesthesia.
- Blood clots forming in the veins.
- Risk in later pregnancies of problems with the placental attachment to the uterus. Women with previous Cesarean deliveries are at an increased risk for placenta previa, a condition in which the placenta attaches abnormally close to the cervix. In some cases, the placenta may also attach too deeply into the uterine wall, so that it cannot be detached after

the delivery of the baby. This condition is called placenta accreta and can result in large blood loss and hysterectomy. This complication is rare, but the risk increases with each subsequent Cesarean delivery.

- Wound separation requiring wound care for several weeks.

The decision to attempt a VBAC considers many factors including how many children you would like to have in the future. One of the benefits of a successful VBAC is an easier and safer pregnancy or pregnancies in the future. If you don't have a desire for future pregnancies, then it may not make sense to attempt a VBAC in some instances.

Breastfeeding

Should I breastfeed?

Yes! Breastfeeding is not the panacea that some people make it out to be, but it is the best thing for your baby if you are able to do it. Breastfeeding is associated with fewer newborn infections, better maternal-infant bonding, lower cost, and greater convenience. There are only a very few reasons why a mother should not attempt to breastfeed, and the vast majority of women who attempt to breastfeed will be successful. HIV was previously one of the most common reasons to not breastfeed, but a recent study states that people diagnosed with HIV who meet certain criteria should be supported if they want to attempt to breastfeed. The criteria that should be met include starting antiretroviral therapy (ART) before or early in pregnancy, maintaining viral suppression, and being committed to taking ART while breastfeeding.

We acknowledge that sometimes it can be a difficult feat and some babies have a hard time with it. Talk to your doctor if you're struggling, find a good lactation consultant, and be persistent. If at first you don't succeed, try again! It can take babies and moms a while to get used to the process.

Also, the old saying "breast is best" may be true, but the rest of that saying is "but follow with the bottle." If, in the beginning, you are not producing milk or only producing a small amount and baby is still visibly hungry after the breast, give them the bottle. But, at the next feed, start with the breast again! The truth is fed is best and whatever is needed to help your baby grow is what you should do.

If you have tried breastfeeding, done the consultations, worked with the baby and tried the tips and tricks but it still isn't working, that's okay! Your baby and you will be fine, and it is okay to turn to bottle feeding primarily. You tried your best and you should never feel bad about that. Sometimes, it just doesn't work out.

I need help breastfeeding.

You're not alone. Most women struggle at some point with breastfeeding. The first few days after birth, in particular, can be challenging. Let's talk about breastfeeding in detail.

Choosing to breastfeed

You have most likely heard of the benefits of breastfeeding. The World Health Organization and the American Academy of Pediatrics, as well as other organizations such as La Leche League, all promote breastfeeding as best for your baby. While infant formulas are safe, effective, and vastly improved over previous formulations, breast milk is superior in that it is usually easier to digest, nutritionally complete, and contains maternal antibodies that help fight disease which are not able to be reproduced in even the best infant formula. Additionally, breastfed babies have a lower incidence of sudden infant death syndrome (SIDS).

Hormonal changes in the mother who breastfeeds are reported to improve healing and slow bleeding after delivery. For some, it is important to know that breastfeeding is less expensive than formula feeding, even for those who purchase a high-quality breast pump. Also, breastfed babies usually spend less time at the pediatrician's office for illnesses due to the passive immunity gained from the mother, especially in the first few weeks to months. Most mothers can breastfeed, and most babies will breastfeed without difficulty. However, there are some mothers for whom breastfeeding may not be the best choice. Occasionally, your doctor or pediatrician may recommend formula feeding if you are on certain medications or have certain medical conditions.

It is generally best to allow two weeks of exclusive breastfeeding to establish a good feeding relationship with your baby. However, as important as exclusive breastfeeding is, it is not the only option. Feeding your baby an occasional bottle of formula or expressed milk after the first two weeks of breastfeeding should be possible. This will allow other family members to participate in caring for the baby and give you a much-needed break. This may be especially important if you have twins, triplets, or any infant that requires extra attention.

What should I expect in the hospital?

Generally, if your labor and delivery was uncomplicated, you should be able to initiate breastfeeding within the first hour after delivery. You should communicate with your health care team your desire to breastfeed and how soon you wish to start. Often, visitors want to come into the room as soon as possible. You should discuss any special wishes regarding visitors with your nurse and doctor. Some newborns are ready to breastfeed within minutes of delivery, while others show no interest in the breast for hours. Offering the breast to your baby in a quiet room with limited visitors is usually more comfortable for the mother.

Your needs will vary, and it is important to be flexible. Some new mothers benefit from one to two hours alone with their infants prior to letting visitors in the room, but this is not mandatory for a successful breastfeeding relationship. It is important that your family and friends understand you may need to be alone at frequent intervals to feed the baby, as often as every three hours and for as long as an hour at a time. You should also remember that you will require some private time for special treatments, medications, or discussions with your nurses and/or physicians.

In the early days, your baby will be getting **colostrum** from your breasts. This is exactly what the baby needs during this time. Most hospital stays are one to two days for a vaginal delivery. In this situation, you will most likely be producing colostrum until you leave the hospital. Breastfeeding your baby on demand will give you the most successful experience. If the baby is awake, chewing on his hands, or rooting (turning his head and opening his mouth), he is ready to breastfeed. It is very common for babies to "**cluster feed**" – where they feed every one or two hours for several feedings and then take a longer four-to-six-hour break to sleep. This is normal. Use these longer breaks to rest or snuggle with the baby. If the baby is healthy, has the appropriate number of wet diapers, and sleeps between feedings, he should be getting enough to eat.

It is very common for newborns to lose some weight in the early days of life. You will notice that the baby has a very dark, sticky stool called **meconium**. Some babies pass stool once a day, others will pass stool with every feeding. Babies are also born with extra fluid stores. Passage of the meconium and extra fluid accounts for the weight loss in the early days of life. If your baby does not lose too much weight too fast and is back to her birth weight by two weeks of age, then breastfeeding is going well. Your health care providers will usually weigh the baby often and alert you to any problems. They will also want to examine the baby. Try to work with them to schedule or allow these exams at a time when the baby is getting ready to eat but not too hungry.

If you have a boy and he is circumcised, you may notice that he is especially tired after the procedure. This is common. Continue to breastfeed on demand but alert your nurses to any concerns you may have.

One common experience is the second night "fussies." At about 12-24 hours of age, many babies will wake up frequently, but fall asleep as soon as they are put to the breast. This pattern will repeat as soon as you try to lay the baby in the crib. Ask the nurses or your support person to help you by snuggling with the baby, offering the pacifier to the baby if you desire, or soothing the baby while you rest. You may also try putting the baby to the breast and gently unlatching the baby by sliding your finger into his mouth to break suction after he has entered deeper sleep. Easing the baby into the crib may be easier at this point.

Special cases

If you have had a complicated labor and delivery, or if your baby requires special care, you may not be able to initiate breastfeeding for hours, days, or, in rare cases, for weeks. It may even become necessary to supplement your newborn with infant formula. You may be concerned about bonding with the baby or how this will affect your breastfeeding experience, especially if you are separated from your baby. In even the most complicated cases, it is usually possible to begin using the breast pump within 24 hours of delivery. Using a double electric pump for 15 minutes every three to four hours will encourage milk production. You will probably express very small amounts of colostrum for a few days (as small as a few tablespoons each day). This is normal. Any expressed milk can be saved for feedings.

When your baby begins oral feedings, these are usually done with syringes, feeding tubes, or finger feedings by staff or parents, and will advance over hours to days to feedings at the breast or by bottle. Try to rest as much as possible and focus on other ways of caring for and bonding with your baby as the occasion allows.

What should I expect at home?

If you are discharged home with your baby within two days, you will most likely not be producing milk. This is normal. By the fourth or fifth day after delivery, you will notice that your breasts are engorged, which means they are full of milk. You may also feel very irritable and cry easily. Often, the baby will have difficulty latching because of the engorgement. It is a good idea to gently express some milk with your hand or massage your nipple until it is soft enough for the baby to latch. Usually, the engorgement will resolve in 24-72 hours. Pumping at this time will only increase your milk supply and prolong the engorgement. However, if you are unable to tolerate the discomfort, you can try pumping just enough to feel better. This will also make it easier for the baby to latch. It is important to remember that this is a difficult, stressful time for some new moms, as they may feel overwhelmed. It usually only takes one to two days before the engorgement has passed and you will be feeling more confident in your breastfeeding abilities.

You will probably also experience nipple discomfort if you are having difficulty getting the baby to latch. Applying lanolin cream to your nipples after feedings, using breast shells to keep your bra from rubbing on your nipples, and avoiding soap on your nipples may help with the discomfort. Finally, your hospital or pediatrician may be able to provide advice over the telephone if you need it. See if your hospital or pediatrician has a lactation consultant or nurse line where you can ask for advice.

Special cases

If your baby was premature, or if you had a Cesarean delivery, you may find recovering at home more difficult than you expected. Try to arrange for help from family and friends prior to leaving the hospital and allow people to help you. Your own recovery, combined with the demands of caring for a newborn, can be tiring. You may have frequent follow-up visits for yourself and/or your baby. Some newborns may require special medications or supplemental feedings. Often, you will have to return to the pediatrician's office several times in the first few weeks. Your pediatrician or care provider should ask you about breastfeeding and provide information and support as well as evaluate the baby's growth, frequency of feedings, wet diapers, and general well-being. You should have a support person present for these visits. This support person can help you remember pertinent information, help, keep records, and notify other family and friends about your and the baby's progress.

Helpful tips

Breastfeeding is a natural process and can come easily to some women while others may need help. Almost all breastfeeding mothers require some type of support and encouragement. Here are a few helpful tips:

- Allow the nurses to help you as much as you need it while in the hospital. You will need at least one hour of quiet time to feed the baby and care for yourself every two to three hours.
- Try to feed on demand. Look for early feeding cues, such as rooting, sucking on hands or fingers, or quiet awake times. Your best success will be if the baby initiates the feeding. Often, these periods will last only 20 minutes, so it's best to start the feeding as soon as possible.
- Most babies are very sleepy in the first 12-24 hours after birth. Try waking the baby every three hours during the daytime if he does not awaken on his own. If the baby is ill-appearing or lethargic, alert your nurse or pediatrician immediately.
- Check for wet diapers and stools. In the first two to three days, it is normal for the baby to have two to three wet diapers and at least one stool in a 24-hour period. Once your milk really comes in or by the fourth day, the baby should have six to eight wet diapers in a 24-hour period. This should reassure you that feeding is going well.
- Before you begin feeding, make sure you are in a comfortable position. It is helpful to have a large glass of water nearby, as you will probably notice that you become thirsty while feeding. Drinking plenty of water is important (usually two liters or more a day).
- Bring the baby to your breast in the hold that is most comfortable for you - cradle, football, or cross-cradle holds are most common. If you are able, you can breastfeed very comfortably in a side-lying position. Tickle the baby's lips with your nipple. When the baby opens his mouth, bring his head to your nipple. Do not stretch your breast to reach his mouth. Most babies begin sucking immediately. Relax your shoulders and arms and rest as much as possible during the feeding. Allow the baby to suckle for as long as he desires. After 20 minutes, if he is still feeding, gently break suction with your finger and try to burp him. Then allow him to nurse on the other

side if he wants to. Some babies will nurse for 20 minutes on each side for every feeding. Some babies will be full after 10 minutes of feeding, but feed more frequently. Getting to know your baby takes time.

- Burp your baby after the feeding by gently patting her back and holding her upright for about 10 minutes. This will also help prevent the baby from spitting up. A small amount of milk may come up with a burp. Sometimes the baby will regurgitate some milk and swallow it without problem. This should subside as the baby gets older.
- Remember which side you started the feeding and start the next feeding on the opposite side.
- It is usually best to change your baby's diaper after a feeding instead of before the feeding.

Do I have mastitis?

If one or both of your breasts is red, tender, warm to the touch, and swollen persistently then the answer is probably yes. You may experience burning or pain when the baby is feeding as well. Mastitis is inflammation of the breast that may or may not have a concurrent infection. Most commonly, fissures or cracks in the nipple allow bacteria to enter the milk ducts and cause problems for mom. Usually, we recommend that during time between feeds you use warm and cold compresses, use Aquaphor or a lubricating agent on the nipple (even dabbing your own milk on the nipple can hydrate the dry skin), and take some ibuprofen or Tylenol. If this does not get better over the next few days or your doctor suspects a concurrent infection, she can prescribe an oral antibiotic that is safe to take while breastfeeding. You can and should still breastfeed with mastitis because it is safe for baby and can reduce the risk of the mastitis developing into an abscess.

When to call your doctor

You should call your obstetrician or midwife if you have signs of mastitis. This is more likely if you have cracked and bleeding nipples and feeding difficulties. These signs include:

- Severe pain in the breast.
- Redness or streaking in the breast.
- Chills and a fever of 100.4 °F or above.

- Flu-like symptoms including malaise, aches, and pains.

Call your pediatrician for questions or concerns, or if the baby has any of the following:

- Less than three wet diapers in 24 hours by the second day.
- Less than six wet diapers in a 24-hour period by the fourth day.
- Refusal to eat for two feedings.
- Vomiting (occasional spitting up should not concern you).
- Difficulty waking for feedings.
- Very irritable or inconsolable.
- High-pitched cry.
- Fever of 100.4°F or above.
- Yellow color of the skin or eyes (jaundice).
- If you think the baby is very hungry or not getting enough to eat.

How do I stop breastfeeding?

The best way to stop breastfeeding is to wean the baby and yourself from the process, rather than stopping suddenly. Stopping abruptly can cause your breasts to get painfully engorged or infected, and the baby may be fussy or not tolerate switching from the breast to bottle or solid food depending on their age. The best way to wean is to start either by shortening feed times or substituting a feed per day with an alternative (bottle or food).

If your breasts are painful during this time, you may want to relieve them by hand expressing a small amount. Pumping instead of feeding will still feedback to your brain to produce milk, so if you must express or pump, do so very minimally so things can wind down. Ibuprofen, cold compresses, and tight bras can all help you during this process.

Life After Birth

Life goes on after you've had a baby. Here are a few things to think about.

How long will my bottom be sore?

Depending on what happened to your bottom during delivery, the recovery time may differ. If you had a spontaneous vaginal delivery and had no tears, the soreness you feel is probably general muscle fatigue and strain of your pelvic floor muscles. This pain should resolve with Tylenol or ibuprofen and a few days' rest. Many mothers feel sore the first few days after, but by their first visit in the office at week one, they say they feel perfectly fine down there.

If you had a tear during your delivery, this is a different story. Depending on where the tear was and how deep it was, you will have a longer healing period.

- If the tear was near your urethra, where urine comes out, it may burn while you pee for a few weeks.
- If the tear was part of your perineum or the posterior portion of the vagina you may have pain with bowel movements for a few weeks.

Any tear and repair that you undergo as a result can take anywhere from two to six weeks to heal. The suture we use to repair that tear will usually dissolve within that time frame as well.

For the most part, when women come back for their six-week postpartum visit, their symptoms from any tears they had have resolved or are close to resolving. Exceptions to this may be a third- or fourth-degree tear, which occurs when the tear extends into the anal sphincter or rectum. Talk to your doctor about how extensive your tear and repair was for more specific expectations of the healing and recovery process.

Why is my doctor asking me about birth control right after I delivered my baby?

We ask because your uterus needs time to heal after delivery, whether it was a vaginal or Cesarean birth. If you want to get pregnant in the future, we recommend that the uterus has at LEAST a six-month period to heal with no pregnancy, with the optimal time frame being 18 months. This waiting period decreases your risk in the following pregnancy of preterm labor, low birth weight, uterine rupture if attempting TOLAC, and a few other outcomes. It also promotes ideal spacing of children so that your first child is independent, becoming potty trained, and less needy by the time the next child arrives.

What birth control should I get?

Great question! For most women, the most appropriate birth control choice is one of the long-acting reversible contraceptives (LARCs). The LARCs include the hormonal IUDs (Mirena, LILETTA, or Kyleena), the copper IUD (ParaGard), and the implant (NEXPLANON). These methods are the most effective (as much as 80 times more effective than the pill), have the lowest side-effect profile and lowest complication rates, and the highest patient satisfaction rates. They also don't interfere with breastfeeding, and they will protect you for 3-10 years depending on which LARC you choose. All of them are immediately reversible if you want to get pregnant, and none of them decrease your chances of pregnancy in the future.

Let's talk more about birth control.

Birth control

There are lots of choices for birth control after you deliver. The choices vary widely, with different efficacies and side effects. We talk about birth control choices in three tiers, with Tier 1 being most effective and Tier 3 being the least effective.

Tier 1

- Intrauterine Devices (Mirena, LILETTA, Kyleena, ParaGard)
- Implant (NEXPLANON)
- Sterilization (female and male)

Tier 2

- Combined oral contraceptive pills (OCPs – "The Pill")
- Birth control vaginal ring (NuvaRing)
- Birth control patch
- The shot (Depo-Provera)
- Minipills (progestin-only pill)

Tier 3

- Condoms
- Withdrawal method
- Spermicides
- Fertility awareness-based methods or natural family planning (NFP)
- Sponge
- Diaphragm

	Method	One Year Failure Rate (%)	Use While Breastfeeding?	Does it Affect Breastfeeding?	When Can I Start?	Satisfaction Rates (%)
Tier 1	Female Sterilization	0.5	Yes	No	Immediately	80
	Male Sterilization	0.15	Yes	No	Immediately	97
	ParaGard	0.8	Yes	No	Immediately	80.1
	Hormonal IUDs	0.2	Yes	No	Immediately	85.7
	NEXPLANON	0.05	Yes	No	Immediately	78.7
Tier 2	The Pill	8.4	Yes	No	4-6 Weeks	53.6
	Patch	8.4	Yes	No	4-6 Weeks	44.3
	Vaginal Ring	8.4	Yes	No	4-6 Weeks	52.7
	Minipill	8.4	Yes	No	4-6 Weeks	53.6
	Depo-Provera	6	Yes	No	Immediately	54
Tier 3	Condoms	18	Yes	No	Immediately	–
	Fertility Awareness	24	Yes	No	After Weaning	–
	Withdrawal	22	Yes	No	Immediately	–
	Diaphragm	12	Yes	No	Immediately	–
	Sponge	24	Yes	No	Immediately	–
	Nothing	85	Yes	No	Immediately	–

When picking a birth control method, ask these questions:

- How well does the method work?
- Can I use it while breastfeeding?
- Will it affect my ability to breastfeed?
- How soon can I start it?
- How well do other women like it?

The previous chart answers these questions for you. Notice that aside from male sterilization methods, the hormonal IUDs are associated with the highest efficacy and highest patient satisfaction rate. This high rate of patient satisfaction reflects a low rate of complications and side effects. The Tier 1 methods in general are the best choices, with the lowest rates of unintended pregnancies, highest continuation rates, highest patient satisfaction rates, and lowest side-effect rates.

None of the Tier 1 methods interfere with breastfeeding. Though the IUDs and implant can be started immediately after delivery, not all hospitals in the United States offer this choice; most women still get them in the office four to six weeks after delivery.

There is a myth that combination birth control pills can't be used with breastfeeding because either they will diminish milk volume or because the hormones will pass through the breast milk and affect the baby. Neither of these things are true. However, because the systemic hormones in the pill, patch, and ring can increase your risk of blood clots, they shouldn't be started immediately postpartum. If you want to take a pill form of birth control, you typically will start that after you are six weeks postpartum. Remember though, the actual failure rate of Tier 2 methods like the pill, patch, and ring is 8.4% per year of use.

Feeling down? Let's talk about it.

A lot of women struggle after their baby is born, and that is completely okay! Even though having a new baby is super exciting, it can also be overwhelming, stressful, and tiring! It's important to distinguish between baby blues and postpartum depression or other mood disorders like anxiety. **Baby blues** are common and get better without treatment, but **postpartum depression (PPD)** can be very serious and usually needs treatment of some form.

Before you leave the hospital, your doctor or nurse should discuss your mood with you. It may be that you are doing great before you leave the hospital and when you get home, some mood changes arise. If these mood changes become overwhelming, you should call your doctor or midwife immediately. You'll be asked about your mood at your one to two weeks and six weeks postpartum visits as well. They can identify whether what you are experiencing is the relatively typical baby blues that should resolve in a few weeks or the more serious condition of postpartum depression that may require medication management or therapy (or both). In rare cases, some women may have **postpartum psychosis**. This is a serious and treatable condition. If you ever have thoughts of hurting yourself or your baby or if you find yourself hearing or seeing things that aren't there, call your doctor immediately or call 911.

Baby Blues	Postpartum Depression
Starts within a few days of birth and goes away with the first two weeks	Starts in the first month after birth and up to a year after
Goes away on its own	Needs treatment
Feeling anxious	Feeling guilty, hopeless, having panic attacks
Crying for no apparent reason	Crying due to anxiety or depression
Feeling sad and a bit off	Having scary and intrusive thoughts
Tired and grumpy	May have thoughts of hurting yourself or your baby

The management for postpartum depression is like general depression. We can try therapy and/or medications. If you discuss medications and decide that you want to try them, it is important that you know there are many medications that are safe for breastfeeding. These medications are usually used for about six months and then reevaluated. Never hesitate to discuss your mood with your doctor or midwife. Together, the two of you and your support system (family, friends, etc.) can come up with a plan to help you feel better.

When can I have sex again?

It depends. Although we classically tell women to wait six weeks after delivery to resume sex, many do not and there isn't really any science behind this advice. The actual answer varies by woman, and likely depends on how you delivered (vaginally or Cesarean), if you had problems (a bad tear or no tear), and whether you have the energy and interest.

Here are some things you should know:

- If you aren't lactating, you will probably ovulate again about 25 days after delivery. This means you could get pregnant from sex that happens as early as three weeks after delivery. Since the time of return to ovulation is variable from person to person, just assume that you are fertile any time after two weeks or so postpartum.
- If you are breastfeeding, you probably won't ovulate in the first six weeks, but you SHOULD NOT count on this. Many women have gotten pregnant while breastfeeding.
- If you had a vaginal delivery with a tear, you may need four weeks or longer to heal before sex is comfortable (and sometimes much longer if the tear was severe or it's not healing well).

So, when should you have sex? When you feel like it and when you feel healed; but make sure you use birth control, or you might have two babies in the same year! Many women have sex before their six weeks postpartum check-up and most of those women have sex the first time at three to four weeks after delivery. It's up to how you feel. It is also very normal to not want to have sex for a while and that is okay too. New babies take a lot of time and most new moms find sleep more appealing that sex!

Should I get my tubes tied?

Many women are sure they are done having children and want to know if they should get sterilized. There are many types of sterilization procedures: some patients have only a portion of the each tube removed or clamped while others choose for the tubes to be removed completely. Women can get their tubes tied through a small incision in their belly button right after delivery, or through a laparoscopic procedure a few weeks after delivery. It's also easy to do this at the time of a Cesarean delivery.

Should you get your tubes tied? For most women, the answer is no. There are two things to think about.

First, **sterilization procedures still have failure rates associated with them**, and the failure rate for many sterilization methods is higher than the failure rates for the long-acting reversible contraceptives (LARCs), like IUDs or NEXPLANON. So, if your main goal is to do the best thing to not get pregnant, you might be better off not getting your tubes tied and getting a LARC instead.

Second, **getting a LARC is much less risky and less costly than getting your tubes tied**, plus most LARCs carry fringe benefits, like better menstrual cycles. A simple five-minute office procedure is better than a day at the hospital and general anesthesia.

Another important issue to think about is how many children have you had and how old are you? Many women under 25, for example, might be convinced that they do not want any more children, but studies show that over time as many as 1 in 3 patients in that age group have serious regrets about permanent sterilization. A patient who receives a sterilization but then decides at age 30 that she wants another child has very few options and none that are inexpensive; however, if she had instead chosen a LARC, she would have had a lower failure rate than many methods of sterilization plus the benefits of better menstrual cycles and easy reversibility!

Finally, most doctors now recommend salpingectomy which is removal of the tubes completely rather than "tube tying" which involves clamping a small section of tube or removing a small piece of tube. Salpingectomy has the benefit of being more effective and potentially reducing your risk of ovarian cancer, but it is completely irreversible. Most women who get their tubes tied don't have the idea of a reversal in their minds, but just know that a salpingectomy is completely irreversible. So, if in doubt, just get a LARC.

All About Baby!

I thought it would be over at the end of 9 months?!

No, no. Now's the fun part! All that back pain, exhaustion, poor sleep, and indigestion has been getting you ready for the exciting part!

How much should my baby sleep?

A lot! Newborns sleep up to 17 hours a day. Eventually this will be in longer sessions, but sleep cycles are not regular until about six months, so expect "naps" of one to two hours which gradually lengthen as the baby becomes more regulated. By the end of the first year, most children will sleep 11-15 hours a night.

Should I circumcise my baby boy?

Circumcision practices vary widely due to different cultural and religious expectations that exist. Medical groups around the world that discuss circumcision acknowledge the same facts surrounding circumcision, but they highlight some aspects for and against circumcision differently to either encourage, discourage, or remain neutral about the practice. Some facts are more relevant in other countries than in the United States; for example, the local rate of HIV infection will make circumcision more or less valuable.

Here we will list evidence-based statements surrounding circumcision in a neutral manner and allow you to draw your own conclusions.

- Circumcision is associated with a lower risk of HIV transmission in HIV endemic locations like Africa. In the U.S., the overall incidence of HIV is so low that circumcision has yet to show a protective benefit, even in populations that are more at risk for HIV, such as men who have sex with men.

- Circumcision is protective against invasive penile cancer. However, the rate of penile cancer in the U.S. is 1/100,000 men.
    - 50% of those penile cancers are caused by HPV 16 and 18, similar to cervical cancers. We now vaccinate against those subtypes with the GARDASIL vaccine.
    - Widespread vaccination with GARDASIL would provide a more protective benefit against penile cancers than circumcision and a reduction in smoking and proper hygienic practices would also help tremendously.
- 3% of uncircumcised males will get a urinary tract infection (UTI) compared to about 1% of baby girls and circumcised boys. Circumcision only reduces the risk during the first year of life and most UTIs are easily treatable.
- Circumcision of males does reduce the risk of transmitting certain infections to female partners: HPV (a cause of cervical cancer), herpes, chlamydia, and syphilis.
- Phimosis occurs when the skin around the glans penis becomes scarred/swollen/painful and is unable to retract. This can occur in about 1% of uncircumcised males. There are also cases of phimosis occurring in circumcised males due to the scarring from the procedure (mainly the Gomco clamp method); however, the true incidence of this is unknown. There are multiple steps that males can take to reduce their risk of phimosis - whether circumcised or uncircumcised. The definitive treatment for phimosis is circumcision.

Known risks of circumcision include:

- Bleeding and infection
- Need for repeat surgery
- Meatal stenosis
- Partial loss of penis.

Other things to consider:

- There is no quality evidence that circumcision reduces sexual pleasure.

- Newborns, of course, cannot directly consent to receiving circumcision, though this is true of many things and parents ultimately have a duty and right to make decisions on behalf of their children that involve their health and safety.

A lot of the claims of benefit and harm regarding circumcision are exaggerated. Most men in the world are not circumcised. The CDC states that in 2010 in the U.S., 58.3% of men were circumcised, but in first world countries like ours, we don't really see significant health differences compared to countries with lower rates of circumcision. Obviously, you may have a religious or cultural preference for circumcision. Discuss these issues with your doctor and decide what you feel is best your son.

How do I care for my baby's circumcision?

First, a few normal things: some swelling is expected and there may be small amounts of blood on the first few diapers. If it's more than about the size of a quarter, let your pediatrician know. It's also very normal for a yellowish layer to form over the glans – this is known as granulation tissue and is part of the healing process.

The best thing to do in the first few days is to protect the healing skin. Use liberal amounts of petroleum jelly (e.g., Vaseline) or a water-based lubricant (e.g., K-Y) over the circumcision with every diaper change to prevent friction. Gauze may be used over the tip of the penis for the first day or two, but make sure not to wrap gauze all the way around the penis itself as this could become constrictive with any additional swelling that develops. If the penis becomes soiled, clean gently with soap and water; anything more, such as an alcohol wipe, is generally too harsh and drying. The glans typically heals fully in 7-10 days.

How often should the baby eat? How do I know if the baby is eating enough?

Generally, breastfed babies eat every two to three hours, and babies taking formula eat every three to four hours. For the first several months, babies shouldn't go much longer than four hours without eating, since they don't have enough stored sugar to "fast" longer than that. Little ones tend to show you they're full by turning away, becoming distracted from feeding, or simply falling asleep. If the baby is still fussing or smacking her lips at the end of a bottle or breast, she's probably still hungry. Babies getting enough to eat will generally have one wet diaper for each day of life up to a week of age, then will level off at six to seven wet diapers and (on average) three to four dirty diapers each day. The doctor will measure the baby's weight at each check-up; appropriate weight gain (typically 20-30 grams per day for newborns) is another good indication that the baby is getting enough to eat.

How should I care for the baby's belly button? When will the cord fall off?

Honestly, don't worry about it too much! Just keep it clean and dry – so if the baby needs a bath while the cord is still attached, sponge-bathe rather than submerge the baby. Another trick is to fold down the top of the diaper before fastening; this keeps the cord from being irritated and helps keep it dry. If the cord becomes dirty, just use soap and warm water to clean it; no need to use alcohol or other agents. If you notice any discharge from the cord (particularly if it smells bad), bleeding more than a few drops, or if the baby cries when you touch or move the cord, let the doctor know. Cords usually fall off by several weeks of life; if it's still present at eight weeks or so, bring it to your pediatrician's attention.

How often should I give the baby a bath?

Pretty much whenever they get stinky! If you clean the diaper area well during diaper changes, babies only need baths a few times a week on average. Bathing too often can lead to dry skin, so pat the skin dry and make liberal use of hypoallergenic, fragrance-free lotion after baths.

Should I immunize my baby? Isn't it better to not give all the immunizations at once?

You should immunize your baby! There are a few very specific conditions when a baby shouldn't get immunizations, and if that's the case, your pediatrician will let you know. That is rarely the case, however, so immunize your baby! Thousands of studies have examined the safety of giving multiple vaccines at once with the overwhelming conclusion that it is safe and does not "overwhelm" a baby's immune system. On-time vaccinating also ensures that babies have adequate protection against diseases as early as possible. Practically speaking, giving more than one vaccine at a time minimizes office visits, simplifies parents' lives, spares babies extra visits for pokes, and saves you from multiple trips in the waiting room where others may be sick!

For more in-depth information online, see healthychildren.org, vaccine safety section. Most importantly, ask your baby's pediatrician if you have questions!

What's the best way for my baby to sleep?

The safest sleep environment for a baby can be remembered by "ABC" – **Alone**, on their **Back**, and in a **Crib**. To elaborate, this means babies are safest in a flat crib (or similarly firm sleeping surface) with only a fitted sheet – no pillows, stuffed animals, crib bumpers, fluffy blankets, extra humans, etc. A wearable blanket, sleep sack, or thin blanket swaddled around the baby is okay.

How can I protect my baby from SIDS?

We're still unsure exactly what makes **SIDS (sudden infant death syndrome)** occur, but the best research we have suggests the best way to keep a baby safe is to place her on her back during sleep until her first birthday. This should be on a firm sleeping surface, free of any loose or soft objects (including blankets, stuffed animals, pillows, crib bumpers, etc.), and ideally in the parents' room until the baby is at least six months old. Avoid placing sleeping babies on couches, armchairs, or other soft surfaces. If you are holding a baby and start to fall asleep yourself, it's safest to put the baby down in a safe place, ideally as soon as you feel sleepy but definitely as soon as you wake up. Research also suggests that breastfeeding babies until six months as well as pacifier use during sleep can help reduce SIDS risk. Maternal smoking is an independent risk factor for SIDS in infants. No recommendations can be made for bedside or in-bed sleepers, and bed-sharing is NOT recommended for any infant.

Why won't my baby sleep through the night?!

Early on, it's not unusual for babies to be awake as much at night as they are during the day; they often don't start to sleep in longer spurts through the night until one month or so. So, until then, time and patience! Afterwards, if the baby is having trouble with night-day reversal, it can help to have more "active" sleep during the day – not worrying if there's background noise, lights on, etc. At night, the goal should be for very calming interactions – dark room, minimal noise, low-volume speech. Most babies are getting two-thirds of their daily sleep at night by three months.

My baby won't stop crying! What should I do?

If you made sure all their needs are met (clean diaper, fed, attempted a nap), you might check their temperature to make sure the baby doesn't have a fever. You can also check to make sure the baby doesn't have any hair or string caught around small body parts (fingers, toes, or penis; these are called "hair tourniquets"). If you've done all of this and haven't found anything out of the ordinary, try swaddling the baby, rocking her, or walking with her, offering a pacifier or her thumb/finger to suck, or turning on soothing sounds (e.g., soft music or white noise, like a fan). If you've tried these things and she is still upset, it is okay to put the baby in a safe place and take a break, especially if you feel yourself getting frustrated. Give it ten to fifteen minutes (or longer if you still feel upset), then try soothing measures again. If crying persists no matter what you do, it might be time to call the doctor's office.

Does my baby have jaundice?

Jaundice causes the skin to appear more yellow, usually starting in the face (especially under the tongue and in the whites of the eyes) then spreading to the chest, abdomen, and limbs. It can also cause the whites of the eyes to appear yellow. If the baby is appearing more yellow than at her last check-up, you notice that her belly, arms, or legs are yellow or eyes are yellow, talk to her pediatrician, especially if she is acting fussier, eating less, or harder to wake up.

Is green poop normal?

Totally, especially in the first few weeks! Depending on whether the baby is breast or bottle fed, stools can be greenish yellow to brown or tan in color, and loose and seedy to peanut butter consistency. Colors poop should NOT be are black, with visible blood, or white and chalk-like. If they are, talk to your baby's doctor!

Do I need to "pump and dump" if I have a drink?

No! Alcohol does pass easily into breastmilk, but it's also absorbed from milk much like it is from the bloodstream. Basically, if you are sober enough to drive, you're likely sober enough to breastfeed. A rough average time to wait is about two to three hours after one drink. If you breastfeed a little early, it's unlikely the baby will receive enough to be harmful. Only a very small percentage of the alcohol is passed on to the baby in breastmilk. Of course, if you had more than one or two drinks and will need to wait longer than usual between feeds, pumping and dumping may make you more comfortable! Also, bear in mind that current research suggests that "moderate" alcohol use (generally meaning less than one drink per day) is not considered harmful to babies. More than that and you could be putting baby at risk; there is no known "safe" amount of alcohol in breastmilk, and some research suggests frequent alcohol use during breastfeeding may put babies at risk for slowed development and poor weight gain.

What's up with my baby's skin?

The good thing is, there are a lot of birthmarks and rashes that babies get, and only a small amount of them are scary! **Milia** and **neonatal acne** are commonly seen on a baby's face and will improve on their own. A splotchy red rash may be **erythema toxicum neonatorum (baby acne)** in the first few days of life or may be a heat rash if the baby was a little over-bundled. Importantly, a blistering rash (i.e., fluid-filled bubbles) might be several normal or benign conditions but also could be a sign of infection you should have checked out by a doctor.

Look at this website for images and descriptions, as well as red flag symptoms of a rash that should send you to the doctor if you see them.

What's This?

Gestational hypertension

This is a blood pressure disorder of pregnancy that is diagnosed by two blood pressures taken at least four hours apart that are $\geq$ 140/90 mmHg. You must be at least 20 weeks' gestation to be diagnosed with this disorder and have no history of hypertension. We will usually not treat this condition with medication unless the blood pressure warrants it, or it progresses. However, we will monitor your pregnancy more closely and deliver you at 37 weeks' gestation (term).

Preeclampsia

This is also a blood pressure disorder of pregnancy that is diagnosed by two blood pressures taken at least four hours apart that are $\geq$ 140/90 mmHg and evidence of protein in your urine. You must be 20 weeks' gestation or more to be diagnosed with this disorder, and your physician will order more labs to determine if there is any associated organ damage or blood problems occurring because of how the disease progresses. Depending on the severity of the disease and when it is diagnosed, you may require blood pressure medications and/or IV magnesium sulfate that helps prevent seizures from occurring. The goal will also be delivery at 37 weeks' gestation unless the disease progresses and warrants earlier delivery for the safety of baby and mom. It you have "severe features," you will be delivered no later than 34 weeks' gestation.

Hyperemesis gravidarum

This is a disorder of pregnancy during which a pregnant woman has excessive nausea and vomiting to the point where she has weight loss, dehydration, and volume depletion that can lead to ketones in the blood or urine, other electrolyte abnormalities, and often an inability to do daily activities. It may require hospital admission and nutrient/fluid repletion within the hospital. It usually occurs in the first or early second trimester.

Gestational diabetes

Between 24 and 28 weeks' gestation, we will perform a glucose *screening* test for gestational diabetes. We will have you drink 50 grams of glucose and then check your blood sugar in an hour. If you fail this screening test, then we will have you take a *diagnostic* 3-hour glucose tolerance test. If you fail that test as well, you will be diagnosed with gestational diabetes. Depending on how your blood sugars are, you may just be closely monitored and encouraged to change your diet and activity level to maintain normal blood glucoses. If your sugars are not well-controlled in pregnancy, then you may need to be started on insulin. Each person will have an individualized treatment plan. Gestational diabetes increases your risk of a large baby, shoulder dystocia at delivery, and Cesarean delivery. It also increases your lifetime risk of developing type 2 diabetes, and the newborn may have low blood sugars at birth and a few other issues which your pediatrician will check on.

Rh negative

Early in pregnancy, you will have your blood type checked (A+, A-, B+, etc.). The + or – indicates your Rhesus (Rh) status. We pay attention to Rh in pregnancy because if mom is Rh negative, we give her RhoGAM (or an equivalent product) near the 28-week visit, and possibly at the time of delivery if the baby is Rh positive. The reason we give this is so the mother doesn't form antibodies to the baby's blood. If mom were to create her own antibodies to the baby's blood, it could cause a fetal anemia and perhaps death in **future** pregnancies if that fetus were Rh positive. If mom is Rh positive, we don't have to worry about any of this.

Advanced maternal age (AMA)

AMA is defined as 35 years or older at the estimated time of delivery. This feels harsh to say, we know! This designation was created in the 1970s to indicate patients who had higher risk of fetal chromosomal problems like Down syndrome and was made as a billing code for women who wanted to pursue testing for these conditions. There are some issues with being pregnant at an older age, but those risks are largely based upon your overall health status, not your age alone.

Miscarriage

Miscarriage is defined as an early pregnancy loss that occurs at less than 20 weeks' gestation. Miscarriages are common and become more common the older you get, ranging from about 1 in 6 known pregnancies for younger patients to 1 in 3 for older patients. Miscarriage can be due to several reasons. The most common cause is a chromosomal abnormality that is not compatible with life. About 95% of miscarriages happen very early, usually before six weeks' gestation.

After multiple miscarriages, there are certain conditions we can test for that are associated with recurrent pregnancy loss. Late pregnancy losses (after 20 weeks) are always investigated because these are more likely to be due to a specific cause.

Miscarriage can be a very disheartening thing, but a single miscarriage does not increase your risk of having another miscarriage! That is very important to know.

Twins

There are several types of twins. The type of twin pregnancy depends on whether it results from one egg or two, and if one egg, depending on when the embryo splits. Twins that result from one fertilized egg are called **monozygotic twins** and twins from two fertilized eggs are called **dizygotic twins**.

All dizygotic twins have two placentas; this is called **dichorionic.** They also have two internal compartments (amniotic sacs) which we refer to as **diamniotic**. Dizygotic twins are also called **fraternal twins.**

Monozygotic twins that split very early will also be dichorionic-diamniotic, but they will be **identical** since they came from the same embryo. However, if they split a bit later, they may have only one placenta; this is called **monochorionic**. Monochorionic twins can also be diamniotic with a dividing membrane between the two fetuses, but they can also have no dividing membrane; this is called **monoamniotic.**

All types of twin pregnancies are at an increased risk for essentially every complication of pregnancy, including preterm birth, gestational diabetes, hypertensive disorders of pregnancy such as gestational hypertension or preeclampsia, and of course more aches and pains and all the other joys of pregnancy. Monochorionic pregnancies, however, have some special risks. These include a risk for **twin-to-twin transfusion syndrome (TTTS)** for monochorionic-diamniotic twins and a risk of cord entanglement for monochorionic-monoamniotic twins. Because of this, monochorionic twins are much higher risk than dichorionic twins and require significantly more testing.

Most twin pregnancies can still be delivered vaginally if the first twin is head down. The one important exception to this is monochorionic-monoamniotic twins; because of cord entanglement, these pregnancies need to be delivered by Cesarean.

<table>
<tr><td>Dizygotic Twins
(two eggs)</td><td colspan="3">Monozygotic Twins
(one egg that splits)</td></tr>
<tr><td>Fraternal Twins
70% of Twins</td><td colspan="3">Identical Twins
30% of Twins</td></tr>
<tr><td>100%
↓</td><td>25%
↓</td><td>73%
↓</td><td>2%
↓</td></tr>
<tr><td colspan="2">Dichorionic
Diamniotic</td><td>Monochorionic
Diamniotic</td><td>Monochorionic
Monoamniotic</td></tr>
<tr><td colspan="2">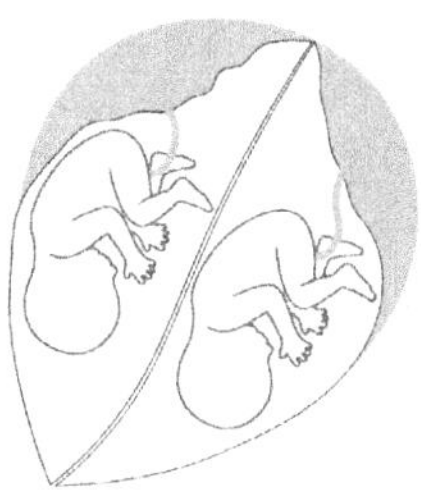</td><td>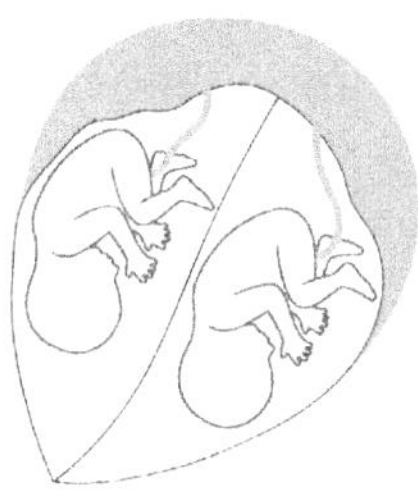</td><td>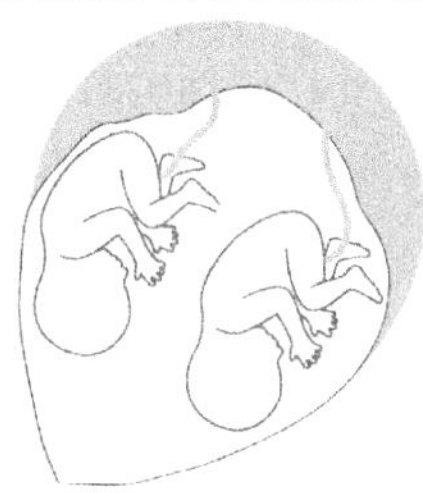</td></tr>
<tr><td colspan="2">No special risks
compared to other types</td><td>Risk of twin-to-twin
transfusion syndrome</td><td>Risk of cord
entanglement</td></tr>
<tr><td colspan="2">Delivered by 38 weeks</td><td>Delivered by 38 weeks</td><td>Delivered by 34 weeks</td></tr>
</table>

MY BIRTH PLAN

Name:

Partner's name:

My delivery is planned as a:

- ☐ Vaginal delivery
- ☐ Cesarean delivery
- ☐ Trial of labor after Cesarean

Before Labor:

- ☐ I would prefer to go into labor on my own rather than be induced.
- ☐ If the baby and I are doing well, I would prefer not to be induced until 41 weeks.

During Labor:

- ☐ I do not want to receive an enema or be shaved.
- ☐ I would like to be free to move around and find positions or places that are most comfortable for me.
- ☐ I would like to wear my own clothes.
- ☐ I am interested in using a labor tub or shower.
- ☐ If the baby is doing well, I would prefer to have intermittent fetal monitoring (every 15 minutes).
- ☐ If I need continuous monitoring, I would prefer wireless monitoring so that I can move around.
- ☐ I would prefer not to have any internal monitors unless necessary.
- ☐ I would prefer to not have observers or students without my permission.

Pain Management:

- ☐ Please don't offer me any pain medications. I plan to use non-medical pain relief techniques.
- ☐ I'll decide whether to use pain medication as my labor progresses.
- ☐ I plan on using IV pain medications.
- ☐ I plan on getting an epidural.
- ☐ I would like the lights kept low in my room.
- ☐ I plan on bringing music to play while I'm in labor.

Delivery:

- ☐ I would like to be able to photograph and/or film my delivery.
- ☐ I would like to have a mirror available to view my baby's birth.

- ☐ I would like to touch my baby's head as I crown.
- ☐ I would like to be coached on when to push.
- ☐ I would prefer to push instinctively.
- ☐ I do not want an episiotomy.
- ☐ I would like to choose the position I deliver in.

Right After Delivery:

- ☐ I'd like to hold my baby skin-to-skin immediately after delivery.
- ☐ I would prefer delayed cord clamping if the baby is doing well.
- ☐ My partner would like to cut the cord.
- ☐ I'd like to delay bathing and other newborn procedures for at least an hour so that I can feed and bond with my baby.

Neonatal care:

- ☐ I plan to exclusively breastfeed my baby while in the hospital.
- ☐ I plan to formula feed my baby.
- ☐ I plan to breastfeed and use formula.
- ☐ Please do not give my baby a bottle or pacifier.
- ☐ I would like my baby to stay in the room with me.
- ☐ I would like my baby to stay in the room with me only when I'm awake.
- ☐ I would prefer that my baby is examined in the room with me.
- ☐ If my baby is a boy, I want him to be circumcised in the hospital.
- ☐ If my baby is a boy, I want him to be circumcised later.
- ☐ If my baby is a boy, I do not want him to be circumcised.

If I need a Cesarean:

- ☐ I would like a spinal anesthetic.
- ☐ I would prefer clear drapes so that I can see the Cesarean delivery.
- ☐ I would like my baby skin-to-skin while still in the operating room.
- ☐ I would like to breastfeed in the recovery room.
- ☐ I want my partner to always stay with me.

Going home:

- ☐ I'd like to leave the hospital as soon as possible after delivery.
- ☐ I'd prefer a longer stay in the hospital.

Anything else:

Notes

Made in United States
Orlando, FL
18 July 2026

84474102R00066